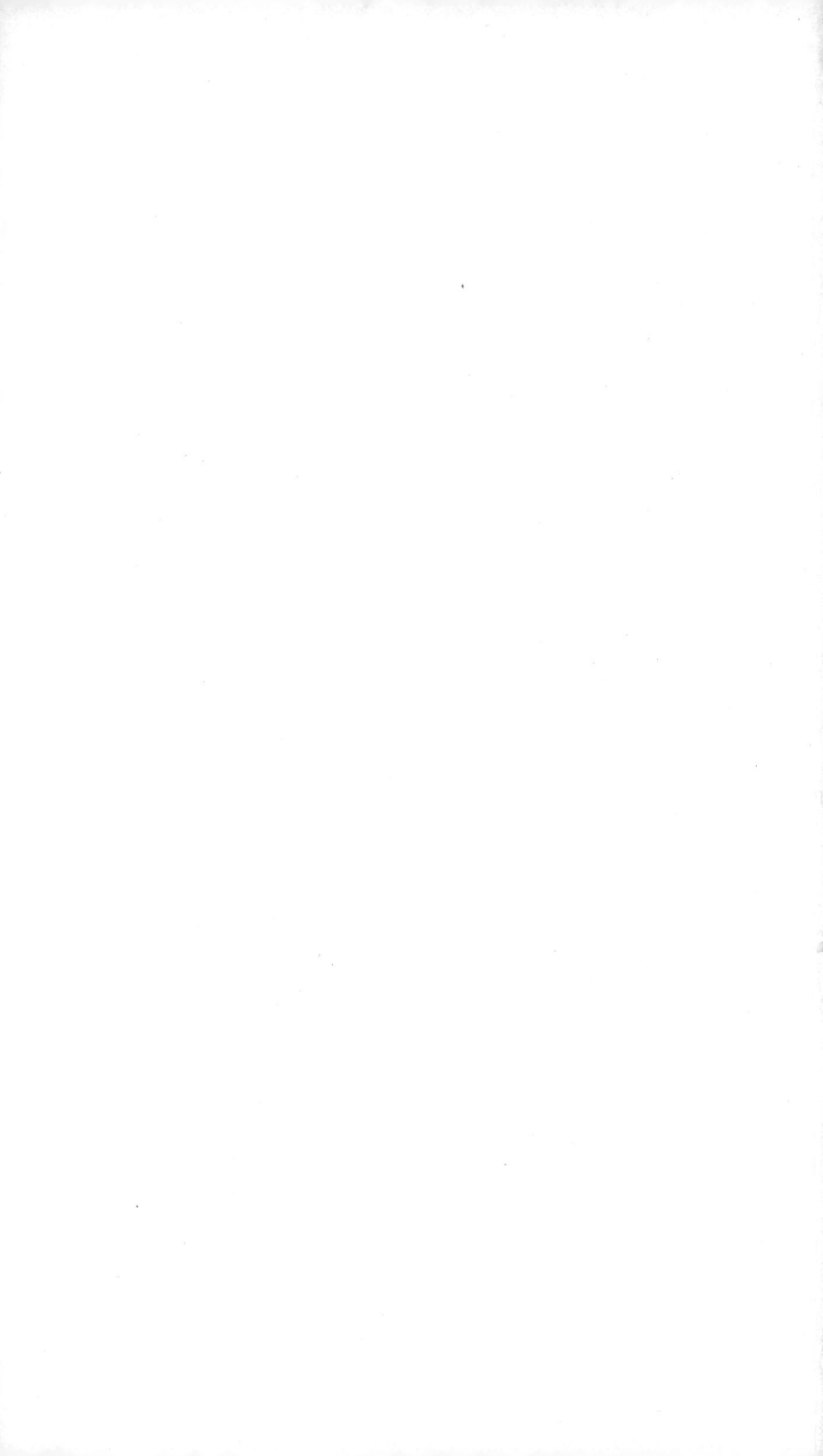

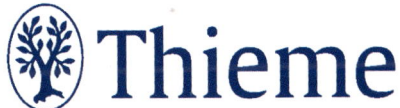

Basics of Vitrectomy

Rajvardhan Azad, MD, FRCSed, FICS, FAMS
Professor,
Zhongshan Ophthalmic Institute Sun yat-Sen University,
Gunagzhou, China

Shorya Vardhan Azad, MS, DO, FAICO (Retina-Vitreous)
Senior Research Associate,
CSIR, Dr R. P. Centre,
All India Institute of Medical Sciences,
New Delhi, India

Brijesh Takkar, MD, FICO, FAICO (Retina-Vitreous)
Senior Research Associate,
CSIR, Dr R. P. Centre,
All India Institute of Medical Sciences,
New Delhi, India

Thieme
Delhi • Stuttgart • New York • Rio de Janeiro

Publishing Director: Dr Sonu Singh
Development Editor: Dr Nidhi Srivastava
Director-Editorial Services: Rachna Sinha
Project Manager: Kumar Kunal
Sales and Marketing Director: Arun Kumar Majji
Managing Director & CEO: Ajit Kohli

Thieme Medical and Scientific Publishers
Private Limited.
A - 12, Second Floor, Sector - 2, Noida - 201 301,
Uttar Pradesh, India, +911204556600
Email: customerservice@thieme.in
www.thieme.in

Cover design: Thieme Publishing Group
Page make-up by RECTO Graphics, India

Printed in India by Nutech Print Services

5 4 3 2 1

ISBN: 978-93-85062-33-9
eISBN: 978-93-85062-54-4

Important note: Medicine is an ever-changing science undergoing continual development. Research and clinical experience are continually expanding our knowledge, in particular our knowledge of proper treatment and drug therapy. Insofar as this book mentions any dosage or application, readers may rest assured that the authors, editors, and publishers have made every effort to ensure that such references are in accordance with **the state of knowledge at the time of production of the book**.

Nevertheless, this does not involve, imply, or express any guarantee or responsibility on the part of the publishers in respect to any dosage instructions and forms of applications stated in the book. **Every user is requested to examine carefully** the manufacturers' leaflets accompanying each drug and to check, if necessary in consultation with a physician or specialist, whether the dosage schedules mentioned therein or the contraindications stated by the manufacturers differ from the statements made in the present book. Such examination is particularly important with drugs that are either rarely used or have been newly released on the market. Every dosage schedule or every form of application used is entirely at the user's own risk and responsibility. The authors and publishers request every user to report to the publishers any discrepancies or inaccuracies noticed. If errors in this work are found after publication, errata will be posted at www.thieme.com on the product description page.

Some of the product names, patents, and registered designs referred to in this book are in fact registered trademarks or proprietary names even though specific reference to this fact is not always made in the text. Therefore, the appearance of a name without designation as proprietary is not to be construed as a representation by the publisher that it is in the public domain.

Dedicated to our mothers
Who brought us in this world,
Our family,
&
All the patients whom we learnt from.

Acknowledgment

To all the staff of operating room at Dr R.P. Centre, AIIMS,
New Delhi who helped us perform VR Surgery

Contents

Foreword

While the Control of Blindness Programme run by Government of India has controlled blindness due to cataract, there has been a rise in the reported cases of blindness due to retinal causes. According to estimates, India is going to be the world capital of diabetes, with 100 million diabetics soon, making blindness due to diabetes a major public health problem in the future. Besides, other causes of retinal blindness, Age-related Macular Degeneration and Retinopathy of Prematurity (ROP) also require special attention. Given this rise in the number of cases of retinal blindness in our society, an increase in the number of vitreoretinal (VR) surgeons is the need of the hour.

VR surgery is a difficult specialty that requires extensive training, guidance and knowledge. These very facts triggered the writing of this book. Though small in size, this book contains a wealth of information that will help those undergoing training in VR surgery. It has been written by renowned VR surgeon Prof. (Dr) Rajvardhan Azad, along with two young, extremely bright VR surgeons who have learnt the art and science of this surgery under the guidance of Dr Azad. In this book, they have shared their technique of VR surgery, which they have mastered.

I am sure this book will fill the void that exists in the literature in the subject despite some standard textbooks and manuals that are available. The beauty of this book is its simple language, and lucid and vivid descriptions through a plethora of images, which reminds one of the saying: "Seeing is like coming out of the tunnel and hearing is just passing through it".

I do sincerely hope that all ophthalmologists, whether budding or blossomed as academicians, and those involved in VR practice, find this work useful and benefit from it.

Dr Balram Airan, MCh, FAMS, FIACS
Dean (Academics)
All India Institute of Medical Sciences
New Delhi, India

Preface

Basics of Vitrectomy, as the title implies, is a handbook for those who undergo training in vitreo-retinal (VR) surgery, either as a fellow, a senior resident or as someone starting his/her own practice in a retina care centre.

Technological advancements have led to a sea of changes in the management of VR cases. Pars Plana Vitrectomy has now not only brought comfort to the retinal surgeon but has also bettered visual results for the patients. However VR surgery is still seen as a difficult ladder to climb and that is why a lot of young surgeons take the alternate path of moving on to specialise in anterior segment surgery.

This book will not only make things easier for VR surgeons to make a head start, but will also enable them to perform surgeries in the best possible manner. The chapters are not exhaustive but they provide all the important information required, and more importantly, the pictorial description of various steps of surgery is aimed at creating a lasting impression for surgeons to make use of inside operating rooms.

While we don't claim any superiority of content in this book, we do feel confident that once you go through it, you will definitely want to refer to it again and again.

We will look forward to your suggestions and feedback.

Rajvardhan Azad

History of Vitreous Surgery

Shorya Vardhan Azad, Rajvardhan Azad, and Brijesh Takkar

1

1 History of Vitreous Surgery

Introduction

History of vitreous surgery dates back to 1863 when von Graefe (**Fig. 1.1**) invaded the vitreous to remove a foreign body. He cut a dense vitreous membrane by introducing

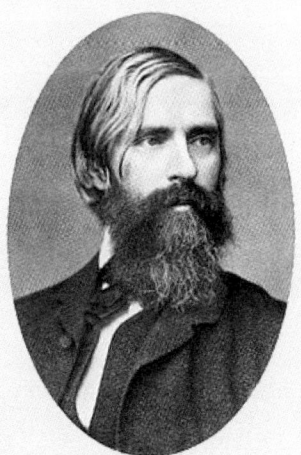

Fig. 1.1 von Graefe.

a keratonyxis needle. From then on, till 1968, there were numerous assaults to the vitreous, albeit mostly fruitless and rarely fruitful. Since then, it has taken 100 years to develop a machine that could cut and aspirate the vitreous simultaneously.

In 1968, David Kasner was the first to carry out an open-sky vitrectomy, which involved vitrectomy through a penetrating keratoplasty incision (**Fig. 1.2**). His first case involved removing the diseased vitreous in a case of amyloidosis. Soon vitrectomy became a common practice for vitreous disorders; hence, open-sky vitrectomy had truly opened the sky for a new era marking the start of the age of vitrectomy. However, credit for closed globe vitrectomy

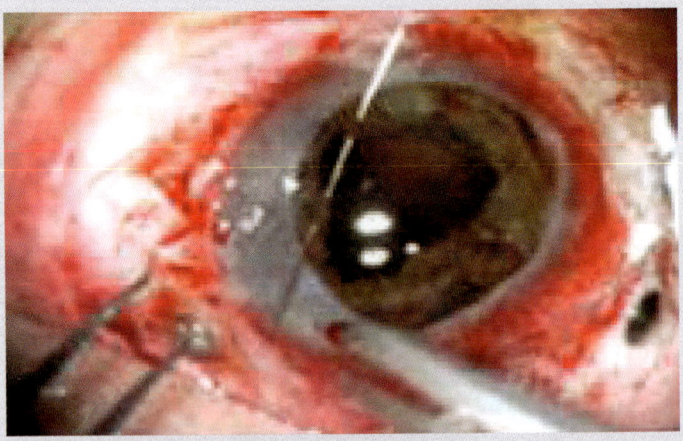

Fig. 1.2   An example of open-sky vitrectomy.

goes to Robert Machemer (**Fig. 1.3**). He popularized vitrectomy with an electric drill with simultaneous infusion and suction, which he developed in conjunction with Jean Marie Parel in 1970. This instrument was called vitreous infusion suction cutter (VISC), and it soon underwent various modifications to finally arrive at its 10th design, which was an 18-gauge instrument. His first patient had vitreous hemorrhage and gained vision from counting finger to 20/50. While Machemer produced a single-port vitrectomy system, it was Conor O' Malley and Heinz who brought about the concept of three-port vitrectomy with 20-gauge instruments, which has been widely used till recently.

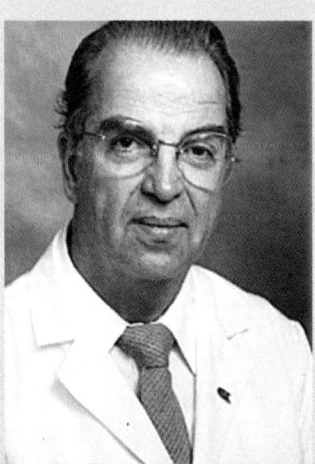

Fig. 1.3   Robert Machemer.

Then started the development of various cutters and machines, mainly pioneered by Rudolf Kloti and Peyman, although in separate capacities. Both of them popularized oscillatory type of cutters, which in comparison to rotating cutters had less chances of tissue entanglement. Another important and indispensable addition was the endoilluminator, which was first used by Machemer in 1972.

Hence, with the beginning of the era of vitrectomy, various vitrectomy instruments, fundus visualization system, latest operating microscopes, and endolaser were invented, with a major share of the credit going to Peyman (**Fig. 1.4**)

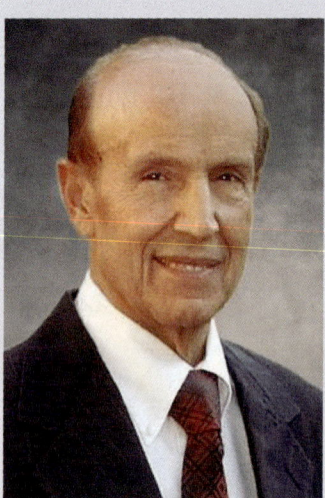

Fig. 1.4 Gholam Peyman.

and coworkers. Another name that needs mentioning is Steve Charles (**Fig. 1.5**), who is credited with numerous additions to modern-day vitrectomy. He introduced the concept of linear intraocular suction device in vitreoretinal surgery. Surgical adjuncts such as perfluorocarbon liquid and dyes are discussed later in appropriate chapters.

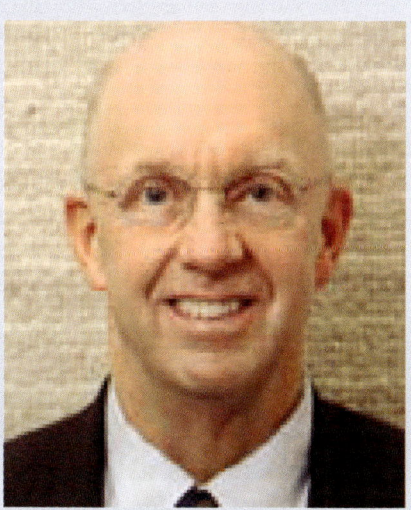

Fig. 1.5 Steve Charles.

Development of Vitrectomy Machines

The first vitrectomy machine was the VISC (**Fig. 1.6**), which later underwent various modifications with better understanding of suction and fluidics required for vitrectomy. However, inventions coupled with advances in technology have revolutionized vitrectomy, making it a very safe and consistent procedure.

O'Malley gave us a new machine, the Ocutome (**Fig. 1.7**). There were some major differences between VISC and Ocutome. The functions of suction and cutting were separated from infusion; the illumination was separated off-axis to improve vitreous illumination; and most notably, the entire system got much smaller, heralding the dawn of the 20-gauge instrument. Ocutome 800 was the first complete system for posterior vitrectomy developed in 1975 and delivered 800 cuts/min and suction of 250 mm Hg.

Then there was notable addition of Millennium (Bausch and Lomb) (**Fig. 1.8**) and Accurus (Alcon) (**Fig. 1.9**), which had cut rates of around 2,500 cut/min and suction of 500 mm Hg.

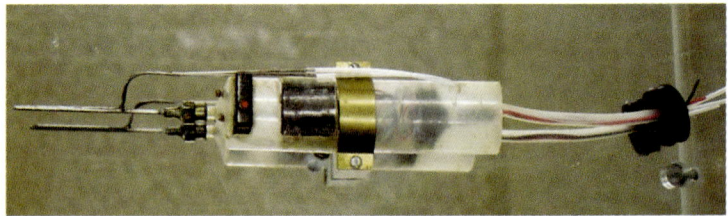

Fig. 1.6   Vitreous infusion suction cutter.

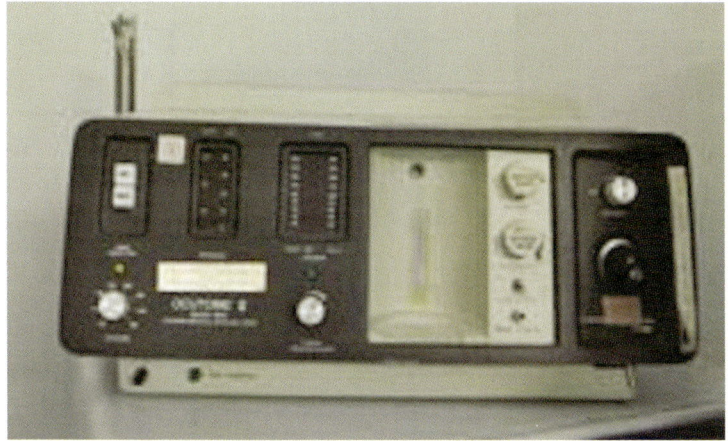

Fig. 1.7 Ocutome.

They also supported minimally invasive vitrectomy systems (MIVS) with 23 and 25 gauge. However, both these systems had separate illumination and laser consoles. Then began the revolution of system integration: a steadily increasing number of functions in one console under unified control using a graphical user interface. Constellation (Alcon) (**Fig. 1.10**) vitrectomy machine, which came next, boasted of integrated pressurized infusion and intraocular pressure compensation, xenon illuminator, 532-nm laser, cut rates upto 7,500 cuts/min with duty cycle control (port open vs. port closed), and auto gas fill. A recent addition is Eva (DORC) which offers 16,000 cuts/min by inculcating a cutter that cuts in both directions. The 27 G system has also been introduced recently.

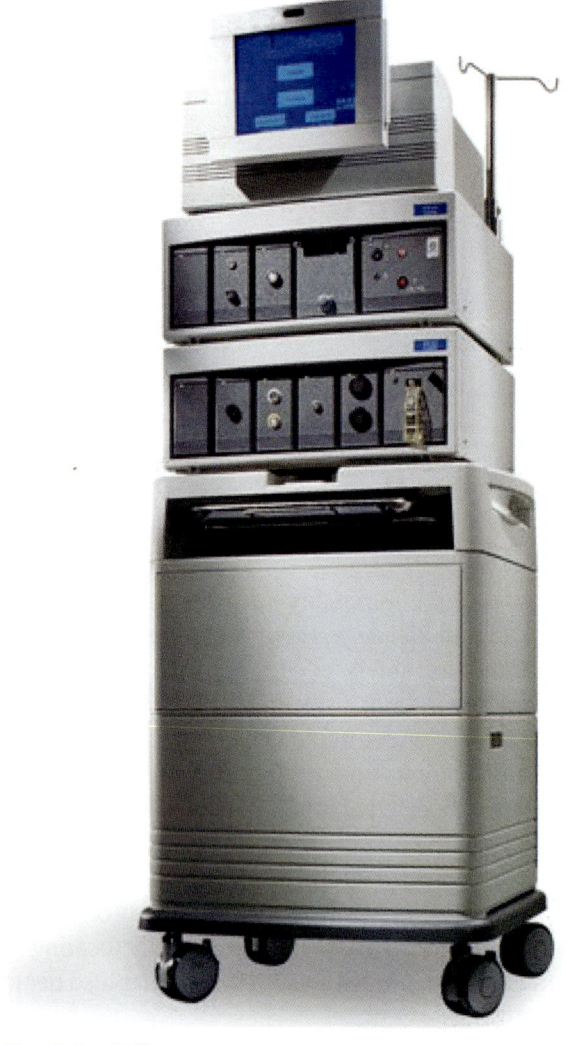

Fig. 1.8 Millennium.

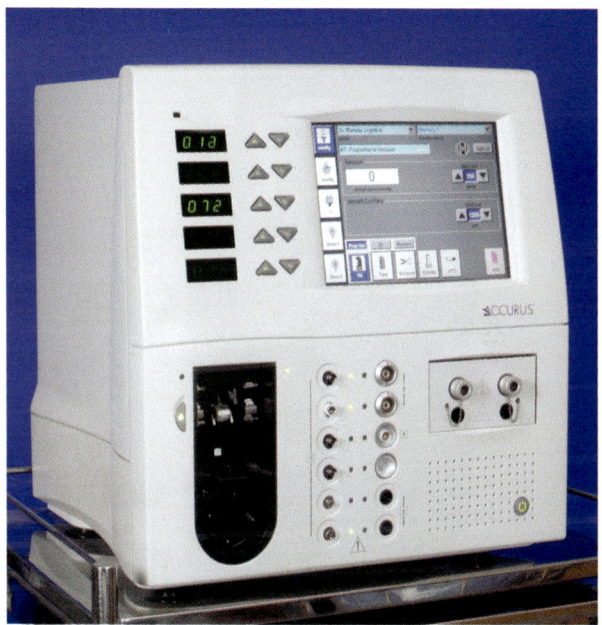

Fig. 1.9 Accurus.

Cutting Technology

After the VISC, Machemer and Douvas developed the RotoExtractor, which, like the VISC, was a full-function, large-incision, rotatory cutter, but incorporated an oscillatory mode to address the vitreous winding problem of the VISC. O'Malley and Heinz developed three-port vitrectomy with a 20-gauge (0.89 mm) system along with a lightweight, reusable, bellows-driven, pneumatic, axial cutter driven by the Ocutome 800 console (Berkley Bioengineering, 1972). Gholam Peyman

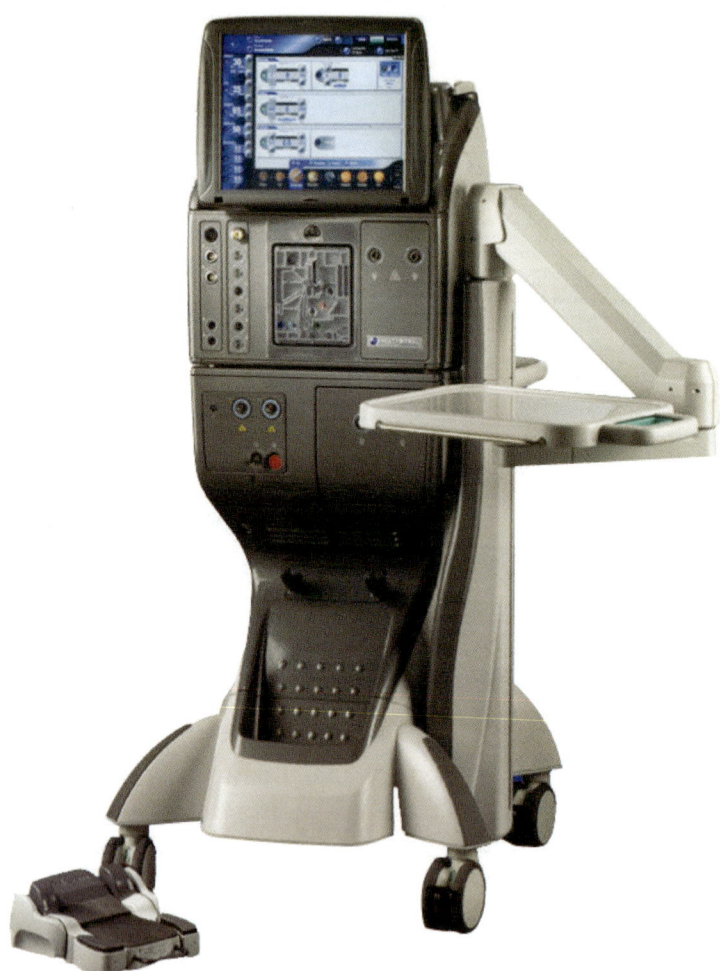

Fig. 1.10 Constellation.

was the first one to develop the electric solenoid–driven axial (guillotine) cutter. At about the same time, R. Kloti in Europe developed a three-port system with an electric cutter. The new cutters, especially the 23 and 25 gauge, have tremendously altered our approach. The improved flow rates and cutting efficiency, as well as rigidity of the instruments, allow us to maneuver and attack tissue anteriorly. Previously, about 20% of our vitrectomies were small-incision surgeries, but nowadays 80% are MIVS. In 23- and 25-gauge cutters, ports are closer to the tip, thereby helping in easy shaving, precise cutting, and aspiration (**Fig. 1.11**). Almost all surgical maneuvers can now be achieved with the cutter, thus making it a multi-utility instrument.

Endophotocoagulator

Steve Charles developed endophotocoagulation to allow retinopexy, hemostasis, and panretinal photocoagulation without corneal or iris damage and adapted the technique to three-port vitrectomy. His first system used the Zeiss xenon source, while his first commercial system used a different xenon source

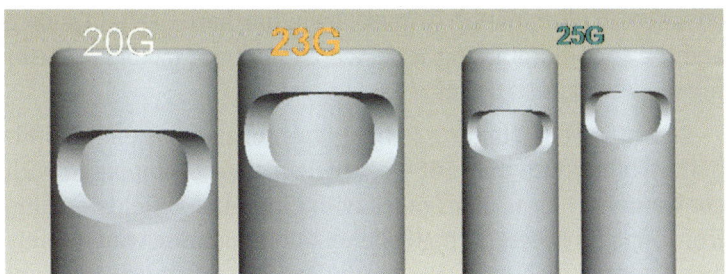

Fig. 1.11 Vitrectomy cutters.

(Patrick O'Malley's Log III photocoagulator); subsequently, Maurice Landers, Jay Fleischman, and S. Charles simultaneously and independently developed endophotocoagulation systems using an argon laser source. Later, Yasuo Tano developed the near-infrared diode laser source, and finally, Alcon and Iridex developed 532-nm, diode-pumped sources.

Endoilluminator

An external slit illuminator outside the eye was initially used in the early 1970s. The current style of endoillumination, using an optic fiber inserted into the vitreous cavity, was first introduced in 1976 by Gholam A. Peyman, for 20-gauge three-port vitrectomy. In the 20-gauge era, a halogen or metal halide light bulb was used as the illuminating source. However, when using a small-gauge optic fiber with a conventional halogen light source, only 50% or less of the brightness found with the 20-gauge system was obtained. To compensate for the insufficient brightness of illumination through small-gauge light probes with conventional halogen light bulbs, improved light sources, that is, xenon and mercury vapor light bulbs, were introduced. Therefore, recent advances in illumination systems, including both the light source and the endoilluminating style, were important factors in pushing the widespread use of MIVS.

Recently, self-retaining light probes (chandelier endoillumination) offer more than 100-degree field of view, compared with conventional "focal" light pipes with illumination fields ranging from 50 to 80 degrees. Chandelier endoillumination would safely avoid retinal phototoxicity as the working distance for light irradiation is as far away from the retina as possible.

Wide-Angle Viewing System

Lens systems for vitrectomy initially employed plano-concave or biconcave lenses, which offered only a 20- to 35-degree field of view. The retinal periphery was difficult to visualize, as even prism lenses could not provide visualization much past 60 degrees. Wide-angle viewing systems were introduced and took advantage of the same principle on which the indirect ophthalmoscope works. Two types of wide-angle viewing systems are available for vitrectomy surgery: noncontact and contact systems.

Contact systems typically provide a wider field of view with fewer aberrations and reflections. However, either a lens ring must be sewn on or a skilled assistant is required to maintain the image quality. Contact lens systems include those produced by Advanced Visual Instruments, Inc. (New York), Volk Optical, Inc. (Mentor, Ohio), and Ocular Instruments, Inc. (Bellevue, Washington).

Noncontact systems do not require a skilled assistant, and they do not cause trauma to the corneal epithelium. Scleral depression is typically easier and manipulation of the microscope foot pedal remains consistent, whether or not the image is inverted. Commonly used noncontact type wide-angle viewing systems include BIOM (Oculus), Merlin (Volk Optical, Inc.), OFFISS (Topcon Medical Inc.), Resight (Carl Zeiss Meditec AG), and Peyman–Wessels–Landers semi-wide-angle viewing system (Ocular Instruments).

Minimally Invasive Vitreoretinal Surgery

*Shorya Vardhan Azad
and Brijesh Takkar*

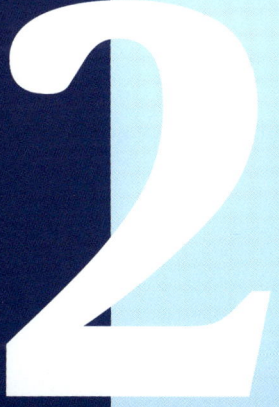

2

2 Minimally Invasive Vitreoretinal Surgery

Introduction

Vitreoretinal surgery has evolved in leaps and bounds with the development of sutureless small-gauge vitrectomy systems. Traditionally, three-port 20-gauge vitrectomy had to be sutured, but now with the advent of 23-, 25-, and 27-gauge vitrectomy systems, ports can be left sutureless, leading to better postoperative results and quicker rehabilitation. Microinvasive vitrectomy system (MIVS) is much more than smaller openings as it has completely revolutionized vitreoretinal surgery.

De Juan was the first to develop 25-gauge vitrectomy system for pediatric use in 1990; however, due to reduced aspiration rate, it was used only in selected cases. Finally, 12 years later, Fuji et al introduced a complete 25-gauge transconjunctival vitrectomy system. Thereafter, Eckardt in 2005 designed the fully integrated 23-gauge vitrectomy with the help of DORC. This combined the advantage of a suture-less system with the rigidity of a 20-gauge instrument that was then found to be lacking in a 25-gauge instrument. The 23- and 25-gauge systems have made surgery time shorter with rapid recovery and lesser astigmatism than 20-gauge system; as a result, 80% of cases are now operated with MIVS. Perhaps, the only indications for 20 gauge surgery now are retained intraocular foreign body, phacofragmentation, and retinal detachment with choroidal detachment.

Wound Construction

It is an important step as it allows the ports to be left sutureless. It is called entry sight alignment (ESA) system as it maintains the alignment between the conjunctiva and the sclera for the placement of cannula. ESA consists of trocar-mounted cannulas (**Fig. 2.1**), plugs, and infusion line. Transconjunctival ports can be made in two different ways: (1) a two-step system in which a trocar cannula is placed after a sclerotomy is made using a microvitreoretinal knife, which was used earlier, and (2) a one-step system where trocar and cannula are sharp enough to make a sclerotomy themselves, which is more common now. This method is also preferred for the reason that the trocar cannula sets are disposable. Newer valved cannulas have emerged, which maintain the intraocular pressure (IOP), hence obviating the need of plugs during the surgery. Insertion of trocar is done after displacing the conjunctiva, followed by 45-degree angle of insertion intrasclerally and then changing direction midway to

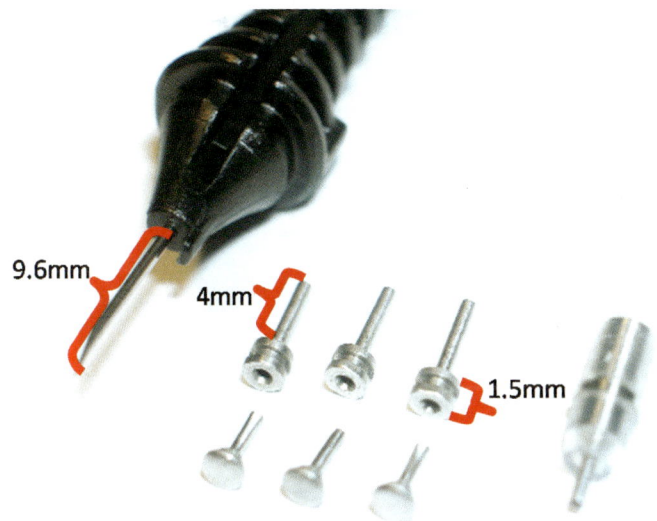

Fig. 2.1 Trocar, cannula, and plugs for microincision vitrectomy system.

perpendicular to give a valve-like effect to the sclerotomy. After insertion of infusion port, cannula should always be checked before starting the infusion (**Figs. 2.2–2.5**).

Flow Rates

Factors affecting rate of vitreous removal are:

- Infusion pressures
- Aspiration pressures
- Duty cycle

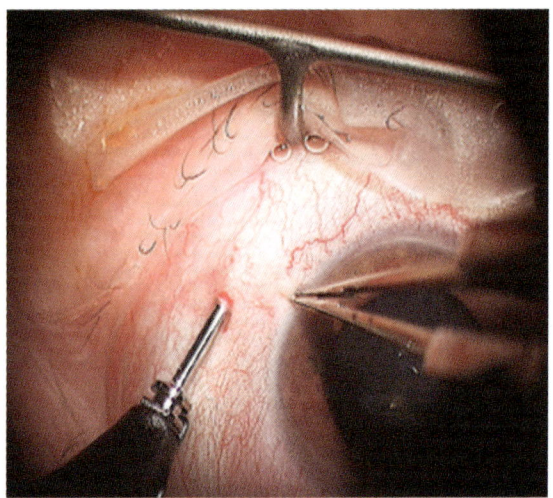

Fig. 2.2 Initial 45-degree angled intrascleral insertion.

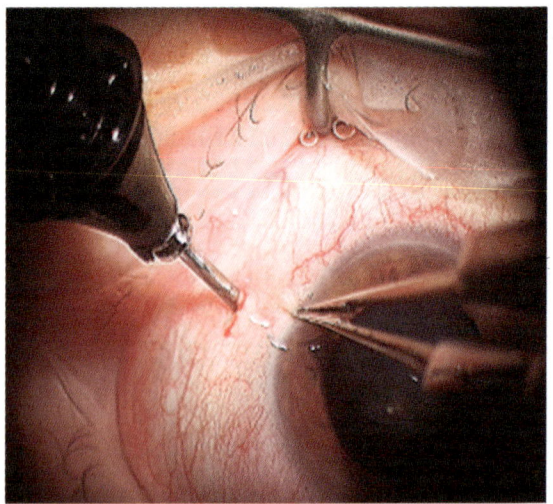

Fig. 2.3 Midway perpendicular shift of trocar for valved entry.

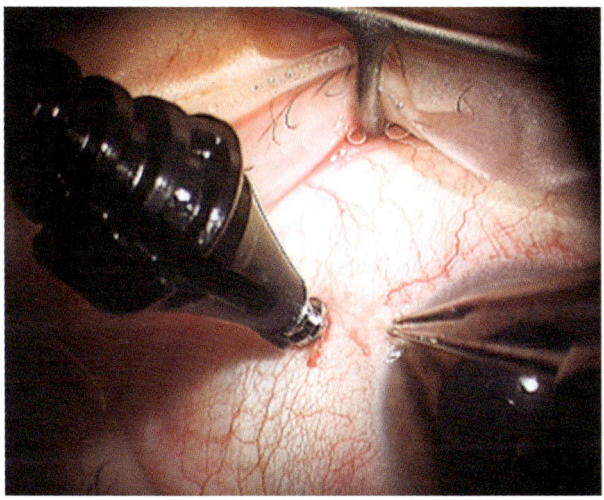

Fig. 2.4 Completely inserted trocar.

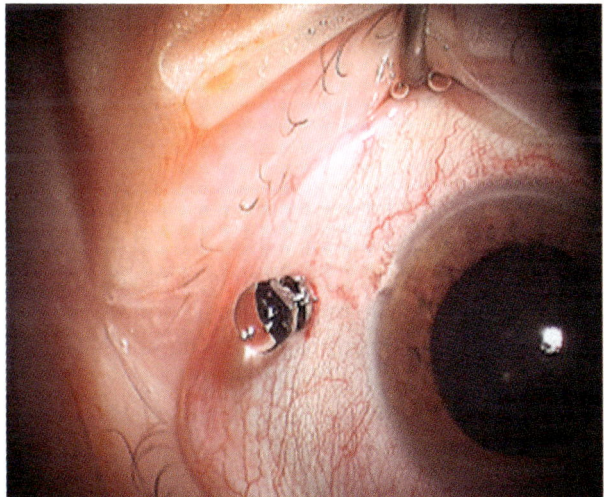

Fig. 2.5 Trocar removed with liquefied vitreous coming out of the cannula.

According to the Poiseuille's law, if we reduce the radius of a tube by half, then the flow rate of an incompressible liquid goes up by 16 times, hence parameter adjustments are required in different gauges (**Table 2.1**). We can use a setting of around 30 infusion pressure in 20 gauge, 30 to 40 infusion pressure for 23 gauge, and 40 to 50 infusion pressure for 25 gauge.

Another important parameter is the aspiration pressure of the machine. Hence, in cases of MIVS, we increase aspiration pressure from 150 mm Hg in 20 gauge setup to 250 to 300 mm Hg in 23 gauge and to around 500 mm Hg in 25 gauge.

Duty cycle is an essential factor which indicates the percentage of time the port is open, measured against the total time of the cut cycle. Normally, with increase in cut rate, there is decrease in the volume of vitreous removed. Some cutters have duty cycles that favor a more open port, while some favor a more closed port, but the new Constellation Vitrectomy System has a duty cycle that can be adjusted to the needs and actions of the surgeon.

Rigidity

Generally, smaller diameter means lesser instrument rigidity, leading to bending/fracture of the shaft of the instrument, which may lead to difficulty in vitreous removal. Traditionally, 20-gauge instruments have been very rigid and stable. 25-gauge instruments were questioned to be lacking and fragile. On the other hand, 23 gauge may actually be the best of both worlds in this sense, having both smaller diameter and better rigidity comparable to 20 gauge. However, newer 25 gauge instruments claim better shaft rigidity, comparable to 23 gauge.

Illumination

Smaller diameter leads to lesser amount of illumination. To overcome this, high-intensity discharge (HID) lamps are used. They are highly efficacious and have a long life.

Complications and Prognoses

Intraoperative

Wound dehiscence: In the setting of recently operated cases for cataract/ globe perforations due to pressure applied during trocar insertion. During trocar insertion, IOP momentarily increases to 60 mm Hg. However, a simple twisting motion during trocar insertion can aid by increasing pressures to only about 30 mm Hg.

Port-site breaks and dialysis: Although reported less in MIVS, they could be present not only at the port site but also elsewhere away from sclerotomies. They mainly occur because of the vitreous entangled with instruments during the multiple exchanges during surgery. This can be prevented by doing a thorough port-side vitrectomy and refraining from multiple instrument exchanges. Port-site indentation also helps in locating breaks in extreme periphery, and proper management intraoperatively leads to complication-free postoperative period.

Postoperative

Hypotony: Hypotony soon after vitrectomy is quite common, generally normalizes early and needs to be managed conservatively.

If not improving, it may require port suturing. It is least common with 25 G.

Endophthalmitis: Although MIVS has received its share of criticism for increased rates of endophthalmitis, recent reports differ as similar rates have been found across 20-, 23-, and 25-gauge systems. In our experience too, rates are similar, although we do emphasize on applying povidone iodine before surgery, as it decreases chances of bacterial contamination from the ocular surface. **Table 2.1** compares the characteristics of the 20-, 23-, and 25-gauge systems.

Disadvantages

- Incomplete vitrectomy especially around the cannula
- Managing anterior PVR
- Subconjunctival oil
- Lensectomy is difficult
- Suprachoroidal cannula
- Intraoperative shift in cannula position

Port Closure

Port closure should be done slowly at a pressure of 20 mm Hg by gently pushing the conjunctiva over it and massaging it. Pressure can be increased after massaging to 30 mm Hg for valve-like closure. Saline should be used to check for port-site leaks and one should not hesitate to suture if required.

Table 2.1 Characteristics of the 20-, 23-, and 25-gauge systems

Parameters	20 gauge	23 gauge	25 gauge
Indications	RIOFB Phacofragmentation RD with CD	All except indication of 20 gauge	
Diameter	0.9 mm	0.67 mm	0.5 mm
Ports	Scleral	Transconjunctival	
Cutter	Port to tip distance more—dissection difficult	Port to tip distance less—dissection easier Multi-utility instrument	
Illumination	Halogen	Xenon, mercury vapor	
Vitrectomy-suction* Core peripheral	150 mm Hg 50 mm Hg	350 mm Hg 100–150 mm Hg	500 mm Hg 150–200 mm Hg
Vitrectomy-infusion* Fluid Air	20–30 mm Hg 30–40 mm Hg	30–40 mm Hg 40–50 mm Hg	30–50 mm Hg 40–60 mm Hg
Rigidity	More	Less	Lesser
Surgical time	Longer	Shorter	
Lens touch	More	Less	
Overfill (oil)	More	Less	
Port closure	Suture	Sutureless	
Post-op recovery	Longer	Shorter	
Patient discomfort	More	Less	
Astigmatism	More	Less	
Tear film	More affected	Less affected	

Abbreviations: CD, choroidal detachment; RD, retinal detachment; RIOFB, retained intraocular foreign body.
*Parameters have to be changed continuously as per the requirement.

Indications and Case Selection

Shorya Vardhan Azad and Brijesh Takkar

3

3 Indications and Case Selection

Introduction

Rapid advancement in vitreous surgery in recent years has led to increase in its indications. With improving skill and exploration, traversing the truth of vitreous has now taken a front seat in ophthalmology from the back of the eye. Mentioning all indications of vitreous surgery in this small compendium is neither possible nor the intention of the authors; the approach, however, is to deal with the important ones.

Common indications of vitrectomy:

- Lens related:
    - Subluxated lens
    - Dropped nucleus/cortical matter
    - Dropped intraocular lens

- Macular surgery:
    - Tractional retinal detachment (TRD)
    - Macular hole
    - Epiretinal membrane
    - Vitreomacular traction
    - Cystoid macular edema

- Retinal detachment:
  - Primary vitrectomy in rhegmatogenous retinal detachment (RRD)
  - Retinal detachment with proliferative vitreoretinopathy (PVR)
  - Combined TRD with RRD
- Others: retained intraocular foreign body (RIOFB)/endophthalmitis/vitreous hemorrhage

This list is not complete, and newer indications keep on adding.

Selection of Cases

The next important step is selection of cases that would benefit most from surgery. Surgical indication depends on more than just the ocular status. Therefore, the aim of case selection should be to avoid bilateral blindness first and then unilateral. It is important for the surgeon to do all the tests himself/herself so as to have firsthand information of all clinical and investigative findings. A good surgeon is one who knows not only when to operate but also when not to operate.

General Status

Age: Among the general status, extremes of age need careful evaluation. Although no age is contraindication to surgery, very old patients above 80 years and young infants are considered high anesthetic risk cases. Early intervention may be required in cases of children as amblyopia remains a concern, while old patients with unilateral disease may not be operated due to shorter expected lifespan.

Systemic status: A complete and thorough systemic work-up is mandatory, including past and present history of any treatment or surgery.

Diabetics: Many patients undergoing vitrectomy are diabetics. Generally, these patients are poorly controlled. Blood sugar profile, HbA1c profile, and urine sugar estimation are essential. It is commonly seen that these patients have poor renal status too, along with anemia, and some of these patients are also on hemodialysis. A close monitoring of blood sugar and renal function is important before taking up these patients for surgery.

Hypertension: High blood pressure needs preoperative control and monitoring.

Infection: Any patient having an infection risk should wait for surgery until it is controlled with proper antibiotics.

Patients with chronic obstructive lung disease and asthma and also those with claustrophobia/anxiety problem should be counseled well about the surgical procedure and operating time. Appropriate consultations should be taken from attending specialist before surgery.

It is always better to discuss the risks with the patient or his/her close relative so that an unpleasant situation does not arise later.

Ocular Status

Visual function assessment: Visual function is a sum total of both subjective and objective tests. Distant visual acuity test is an important tool to assess visual function. Usually the vision is quite low in these patients undergoing vitrectomy; hence, testing for hand movement, projection of rays, and perception of light should be done with utmost care. When perception of light is in question, it must be repeated several times before decision making. In dense vitreous hemorrhage, thick membranes and opaque media torch, light should be at maximum, or a brighter source of light should be used in dark room while assessing projection of rays.

Intraocular pressure: Intraocular pressure (IOP) is very important as it may indirectly give a hint regarding angle neovascularization. Low IOP on tonometry is an indication of associated retinal detachment or an eye going into phthisis bulbi with ciliary body atrophy. Raised IOP can also be present in cases of Schwartz syndrome and associated trauma.

Corneal status: This is important from the point of view of clarity of media during surgery. A patient having advanced corneal opacity would hinder the view of posterior segment. In case of aphakes and repeated surgeries, specular count should be done.

Anterior segment: Preoperatively, the surgeon must have an idea about the extent of pupillary dilatation in a given case as this has a direct effect on patient's surgery. In patients with diabetes, aphakia, and Marfan syndrome, small pupil is a known phenomenon. Detection of rubeosis iridis is important as it indicates the severity of an ischemic process.

Pupillary reaction: It is a measure of optic nerve function; however, involvement of iris in diabetic patients limits its value.

Lenticular opacity: This is another limiting factor. An assessment of the amount of lenticular opacity helps the surgeon to decide whether lens removal is required or not in a given case. It is important to remember the hardness of lens in an older age group. A subjective assessment of nuclear sclerosis helps in deciding which case would require phacoemulsification or pars plana lensectomy. Macular cases should always be done after clearing the media completely as even a small posterior subcapsular cataract might be a hindrance.

Vitreous and Retina

Indirect ophthalmoscopy: Examination by both indirect ophthalmoscopy and slit lamp biomicroscopy with +90D gives a complete view of retinal topography. This examination is also very useful because it provides stereopsis, wide field, and greater penetration in hazy media. Attempts should be made to look into the vitreous changes in the form of degeneration, organized membrane, fresh blood, and any peripheral area of retinal detachment.

Retinal pathology: A proper documentation of retinal lesions is a must before taking on vitreous surgery. A drawing of retinal lesion with respect to the following is mandatory:

- Posterior vitreous detachment (PVD) should be assessed as it is an important step during surgery.

- Retinal breaks: the location, size, edges everted or normal, number of breaks, retinal tear with traction but without PVR changes, and retinal tear with PVR changes.

- Retinal detachment: An idea regarding the nature of retinal detachment, that is, pure traction detachment or combined traction and RRD or pure RRD, should be made as it helps in planning the surgery.

- Retinal neovascularization: Information such as location, size, and extent (both anterior and posterior) is very important (flat/raised).

- Preretinal membrane: Area and extent involved, whether in macula or peripherally situated, and color of the membrane give an idea regarding its origin.

Hazy Media

Macular function: Preoperative vision is the best indicator of postoperative vision. Maddox rod, color discrimination, entoptic phenomenon, and photostress test can be done. Laser interference fringes are also used . However, in very dense cataract and opaque media, the fringes are not appreciated, thereby reducing its value. Therefore, all these tests have limited value and cannot be used as standard tests for visual function, in such cases.

Ultrasonography: It gives real-time imaging and informs us of vitreous motility. Gray scale imaging, on the B-scan, helps us to know about the consistency of the vitreous membrane, whether it is a thin, fragile, translucent membrane or thick, organized membrane, depending upon the brightness of echo on ultrasound screen. B-scan is helpful in delineating vitreous pathology from retinal pathology, condition of hyaloid face (both anterior and posterior), namely, incomplete and complete PVD. B-scan also helps in detecting traction retinal detachments and subretinal bleeds whose view is obscured for example, by dense vitreous hemorrhages. It also informs us about the presence of associated choroidal detachment.

Electrophysiology: In a dense vitreous hemorrhage, electroretinography may be fallacious; therefore, instead of conventional electroretinogram (ERG), bright flash ERG has been in use. Foreign body may also be localized. In bright ERG, the light source is strong and permits the recording of electrical activity of retina. Visual evoked potential can be done in children and in patients with inaccurate projection of rays (PR), as it helps in deciding for surgery.

Therefore, decision to operate or not should always be taken on the basis of simultaneous reading of ultrasound sonography and electrophysiology.

CT scan/X-ray: It is mandatory in cases of trauma, to rule out fracture, or in removing retained intraocular foreign bodies.

Basics of Pars Plana Vitrectomy

Brijesh Takkar and Shorya Vardhan Azad

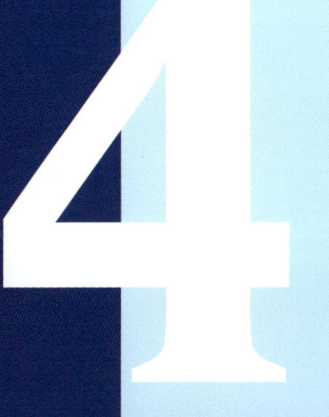

4

4 Basics of Pars Plana Vitrectomy

Introduction

The currently used vitrectomy systems have been structured after a long process of evolution, and are much more safer and quicker. In fact, new indications for vitrectomy are now being realized with the modern vitrectomy machines. Although a general surgical algorithm can be defined, it is advisable that the surgeon individualizes the approach according to the anatomy of each case. This may increase the surgical time, but would definitely decrease the complications and improve the visual outcomes.

Sclerotomy and the Infusion Cannula

Distance of the sclerotomy from the limbus depends upon the lens status of the patient; the distances commonly chosen for the phakic, pseudophakic, and aphakic patients, respectively, are 4, 3.5, and 3 mm. The infusion cannula site is generally chosen to be inferotemporal because of better access and also freedom of movement to the cannula itself during rotation of the eye. The site is advised to be just below the horizontal meridian below the inferior border of the lateral rectus. In the presence of choroidal detachments and in cases like endophthalmitis, the site may be varied accordingly. Once the cannula has been introduced through the sclerotomy, it is very important to confirm the correct position of the tip of the cannula to avoid complications. The surgeon should then secure the cannula with an artery clamp or a surgical tape (while allowing a loop) to avoid inadvertent dislodgement of the cannula from the sclerotomy site. Once the correct positioning of the cannula tip in the vitreous cavity is confirmed, the infusion may be started, as a firm globe allows easier creation of further sclerotomies. The intraocular pressure (IOP) may be set depending upon the gauge of vitrectomy system being used. Lower IOPs should be selected in general anesthesia cases and in those with compromised optic nerve head.

It is advised to make the nasal sclerotomy first, as a high nasal bridge often makes manipulation difficult and it is better to select the most easily approached site of entry and modify the temporal opening accordingly. There is no dictum for fixed clock hour–based creation of sclerotomy sites; however, one may choose to make the nasal opening on the line joining the highest point of nasal bridge and the pupil center, while the temporal opening is on the line joining the lowest point on the superior orbital rim and the pupillary center.

Vitrectomy and Posterior Vitreous Detachment Induction

The choice of vitrectomy parameters depends on the case, the vitrectomy machine being used, and the surgeon's comfort. Generally, one should remember that core vitreous removal should be done at higher suction, while peripheral vitrectomy should be done at the lowest possible suction to avoid iatrogenic complications. Cut rate should be the highest possible for safety. While dealing with dropped lens matter or thick membranes, the surgeon may need to increase the suction and decrease the cut rate, and conversely, while performing retinectomies, lowest suction and highest cut rate should be selected.

Initially, meticulous port site vitrectomy must be performed to avoid port-related complications, although they are now a rarity due to microincision vitrectomy surgery. This is extremely important in cases requiring extensive instrumentation such as diabetic vitrectomies, phacofragmentation, and foreign body removal. The next step is judging if the anterior hyaloid needs to be removed. This should be done when the anterior vitreous cortex is opaque or when there is extensive proliferative vitreoretinopathy (PVR)/new vessels. It is easy to perform in pseudophakia, but in phakic patients, careful maneuvering should be done by gentle aspiration first, followed by safe vitrectomy. In some cases, lensectomy may be required, and if so, the surgeon may use the cutter itself for young patients without nuclear sclerosis or may employ the phacofragmatome. The posterior capsule should be completely removed to prevent postoperative proliferations and anterior PVR. A central opening must be made in the anterior capsule, which prevents postoperative media opacification and at the same time allows for easy positioning of intraocular lens as a secondary procedure. While performing the lensectomy, low cut rates and high suction should be used.

This is followed by the removal of centrally formed vitreous. At this time, the cutter port should always be facing the surgeon to avoid iatrogenic complications, and the endoilluminator should be carefully directed. The surgeon can visualize as much vitreous as allowed by the illumination source, thus highlighting the importance of the "other hand." Core vitreous dissection may be performed under a viewing system most comfortable to the surgeon.

In cases where posterior vitreous detachment (PVD) induction is planned, beginners should always use triamcinolone acetate to stain the cortical vitreous. High magnification and better stereopsis make plano-concave lens the best viewing system for the same. This should be done over both the optic nerve head and the macula. Aspiration of the free triamcinolone is done. The posterior hyaloid is typically engaged nasal to the disc first to avoid macular complications. This is followed by engagement of the superior and inferior cortex at the disc and the macular cortex at the last. One must remember to be extremely careful as macular tears can occur. It is advisable to use soft-tipped cannulas, but the cutter itself may be employed for PVD induction. In cases with adherent hyaloid, one may use forceps to initiate the PVD. Once the Weiss ring is visible and induction over the posterior pole has been adequately achieved, the surgeon may choose to shift over to a wide-angle system and then complete the induction quadrant by quadrant using aspiration with the cutter.

Peripheral dissection is most notorious for iatrogenic complications. After optimization of the parameters, a meticulous clock hour–based peripheral vitrectomy should be done. One must engage the posterior vitreous first and let the vitreous move to the cutter rather than making jerky movements. In phakic patients, vitrectomy across the globe should not be done to avoid the risks of touching the lens. Scleral indentation may be done if needed. If complete vitrectomy is needed, vitreous base shaving should also be done. After this, epiretinal membrane removal, internal limiting membrane peeling, retinotomies, perfluorocarbon injection, delamination, subretinal band removal, and so on are performed as required by the case.

Fluid–Air Exchange and Endolaser

If a fluid–air exchange is planned, one should first place the instrument, mostly soft-tipped active extrusion cannulas, in the subretinal space before switching on to air in cases of retinal detachments. Otherwise, the instrument may be placed posteriorly nasal to the disc in attached retinas. Other instruments that may be used include the *backflush* or the cutter itself. Then air should be switched on and extrusion must be performed. Finally, the exchange can be completed using passive soft-tipped cannulas over the retinotomy/break site.

If laser/cryoretinopexy is required, this is the best time to perform it, as the air allows a wider field and the retinal attachment allows for better laser uptake. A careful indentation of the peripheral retina must always be performed to look for missed/iatrogenic breaks. Green laser or diode laser is usually used. It is important to have the filters in place and keep them switched on. Minimum power should be used and grayish-white burns should be the end point of laser. Power should be titrated and slowly increased. Repeat mode is the best as it allows for minimal burn. The surgeon should keep the laser probe at an adequate distance from the retina, as too far a probe would lead to bigger spot sizes and too near a probe has the risk of retinal touch.

Sometimes, laser reaction may not be adequate despite high powers and continuous modes. In such moments, the surgeon should look for residual subretinal fluid, retinal traction, and retinal edema, and manage accordingly. Although debated, prolonged exposure to air can "air dry" the retina and cause the laser uptake to be poor.

Tamponade

If silicone oil tamponade is planned, the surgeon should remember to decrease the IOP as the vitreous cavity gets filled with the tamponading agent to preserve the optic nerve head perfusion. Careful precautions should be taken in aphakic patients to prevent oil in the anterior chamber and to avoid "overfill"-related glaucoma. Usually, adequate fill is just achieved when the oil is seen to backtrack inside the infusion cannula, at which stage the oil injection should be stopped and the cannula clamped. If gas tamponade is planned, one should remember to use low and constant suction for complete air removal and adequate gas concentration. Thereafter, the sclerotomy sites are closed and checked for leaks. The infusion cannula should be removed last, and before its removal the IOP should be confirmed for one last time by tactile touch, as after its removal IOP alteration is not possible. Whichever anterior segment manipulation is required to be performed, it must be done before the infusion cannula is removed. Sutures may be used if leakage is persistent and is always done for 20 gauge surgery.

Such a surgical algorithm should be kept in mind as it allows for a complication-free surgery. But, as the experience adds on, the surgeon should change the algorithm in accordance with the individual patient to achieve the best possible results.

Vitreous Hemorrhage and Tractional Retinal Detachment

*Shorya Vardhan Azad
and Brijesh Takkar*

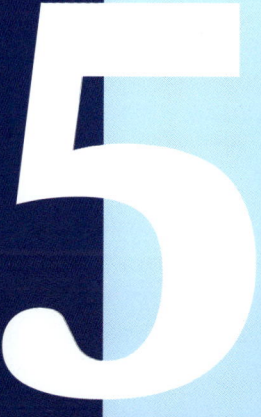

5

5 Vitreous Hemorrhage and Tractional Retinal Detachment

Introduction

Vitrectomy in an uncomplicated vitreous hemorrhage is very rewarding and good practice for beginners. Although earlier one would wait for at least 3 months for the hemorrhage to resolve, with the advancements in vitreous surgery, the wait is now reduced to 6 weeks, with very good results of an early surgery. Many of the vitreoretinal disorders present with a combination of vitreous hemorrhage and underlying tractional retinal detachment (TRD). This is a common manifestation in certain stages of proliferative diabetic retinopathy and proliferative retinopathy such as Eales' disease, and some cases of branch retinal vein occlusion. In contrast, posterior vitreous detachment (PVD) related, traumatic, breakthrough bleed, and ruptured arterial macroaneurysm-associated vitreous hemorrhage do not have an underlying TRD.

Preoperative Assessment

A complete systemic work-up and a meticulous clinical examination is necessary to prognosticate each case. Pupillary reflexes are very important, especially in cases of trauma to rule out optic nerve damage. Macular function tests such as Maddox rod, color discrimination, entoptic phenomenon, and photostress test can be done. Basic laboratory investigations are also necessary, especially in cases of Eales' disease and diabetic retinopathy. Anterior segment evaluation is a must to rule out rubeosis iridis, which might need comprehensive endolaser and intracameral Avastin during the surgery. While significant lenticular opacity requires phacoemulsification, in cases of macular pathologies even a minimal posterior subcapsular cataract should be removed. In cases of dense retrolenticular bleed, clear lens extraction should be considered. Indirect ophthalmoscopy of the fellow eye is a very useful tool for diagnosis. Ultrasonography is the most useful diagnostic and prognostic tool. Fresh vitreous hemorrhage has very low reflectivity on ultrasound, while older hemorrhage tends to form a membrane that demonstrates varying reflectivity. Vitreous hemorrhage may or may not be associated with posterior vitreous separation. A PVD in the presence of vitreous hemorrhage is seen as a freely mobile membranous echo with variable attachments to the optic nerve head or retina. These attachments could be focal or broad, single or multiple. Subhyaloid hemorrhage may be identified as reflective dot echoes posterior to the PVD. The points of adhesion may be associated with TRD or a retinal tear may be identified at the point of attachment. Splitting of the posterior cortical vitreous may also be identified, and this is seen mostly in vascular retinopathies such as diabetic retinopathy and Eales' disease. In addition, subretinal bleed/mass lesion should be ruled out by ultrasonography. Introduction and use of anti-vascular endothelial growth factor (anti-VEGF) drugs has proven beneficial for the complex situations of TRDs, where the fibrovascular proliferations are predominantly vascular. Using Anti-VEGF drugs 3 to 5 days before the vitreoretinal procedure decreases the intraoperative hemorrhage and allows an easier dissection of tissue with minimal bleeding. Similarly, preoperative laser should be attempted whenever possible as it also decreases the risk of bleeding.

There are three goals of surgery:

1. Removal of all media opacities such as vitreous hemorrhage.
2. Removal of all tractional fibrovascular proliferations and reattachment of the macula.
3. Stabilization of the disease process by a good endolaser ablation.

Although vitrectomy in cases with vitreous hemorrhage is beneficial, caution should be taken in the presence of the following conditions:

1. Pale disk
2. Macular ischemia
3. Burnt-out proliferative diabetic retinopathy
4. TRD with extensive fibrovascular proliferation

Surgery

Both 20-gauge pars plana vitrectomy and microinvasive vitrectomy surgery (MIVS) can be done, although now MIVS is the more preferred technique. Ports are made as for any routine surgery. Before swithching the fluid on in cases with hazy media, presence of canula the vitreous cavity should be confirmed by using oblique illumination of the light pipe and the canula mildly depressed with manual indentation. It, however, may not always be visible.

Vitrectomy is initiated by careful removal of the hemorrhage in the retrolental area; special care has to be exercised in a phakic eye to avoid touching the lens. Any vitreous gel sticking at the back of the lens can be first pulled down with suction and then cut meticulously by avoiding touching the lens. A moderate cut rate with high suction is safe and adequate for removal of even thick and organized vitreous hemorrhage.

Once the anterior vitreous and middle vitreous are removed, it is advisable to look for an avascular membrane (e.g., hyaloid). After creating an opening in the superonasal area (**Fig. 5.1**), suction should be applied in this membrane away from posterior pole to allow any retrohyaloid blood to be removed, which aids in better visualization of the retina below (**Fig. 5.2 A–C**). This is the best time to assess for TRDs and focal attachments of vitreous with retina, which require special care as described later in the chapter.

In cases with simple vitreous hemorrhage, this opening in the detached posterior hyaloid can then be extended toward the periphery (**Fig. 5.3**) and carefully toward the posterior pole. If the posterior hyaloid is not detached, it can be gently lifted off from its attachment at the disk either with or without staining with triamcinolone acetate crystals. Higher suction levels can cause breaks in the retina and hence should be avoided.

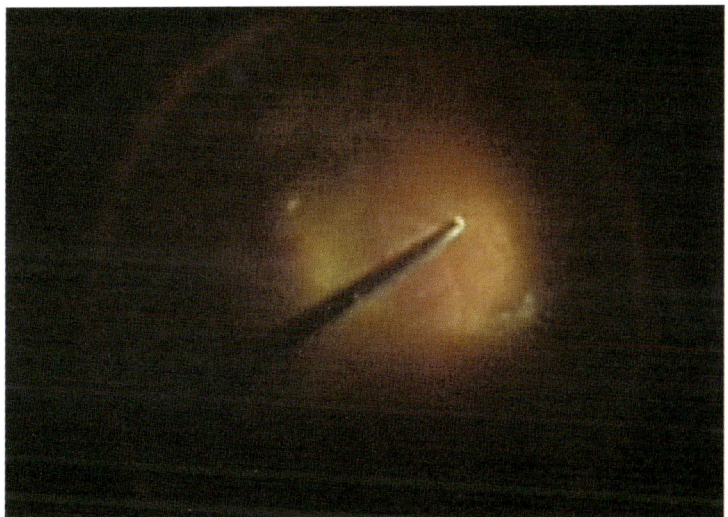

Fig. 5.1 An opening is created in the superonasal area.

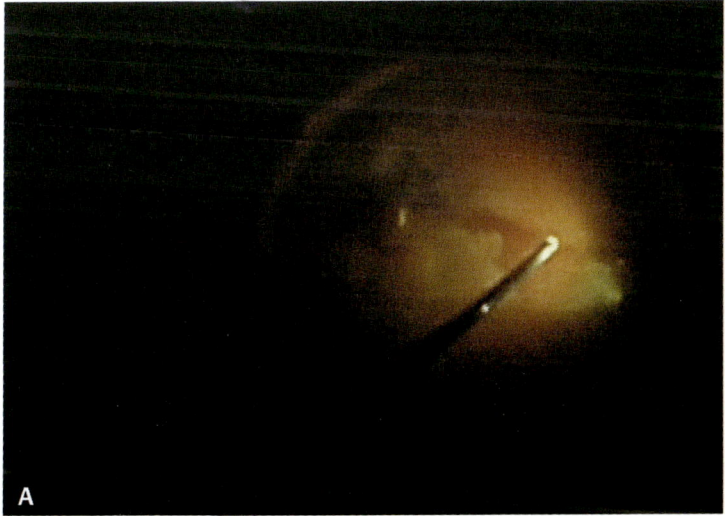

Fig. 5.2 **(A)** Suction is done to create better visualization.

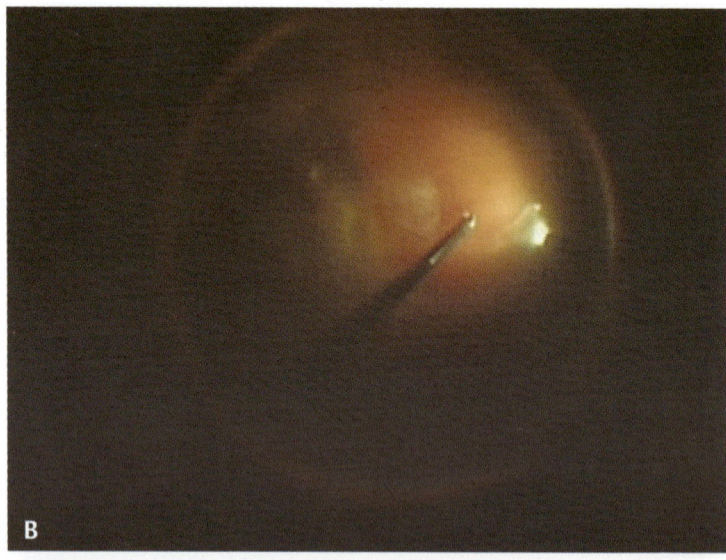

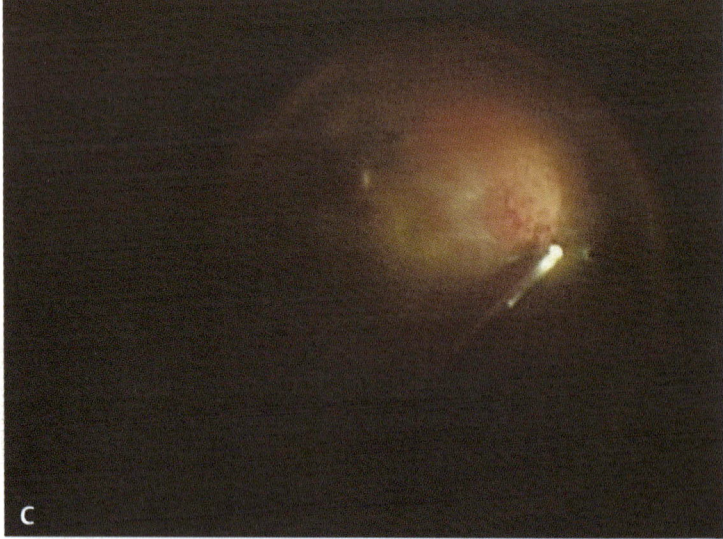

Fig. 5.2 **(B–C)** Suction is done to create better visualization.

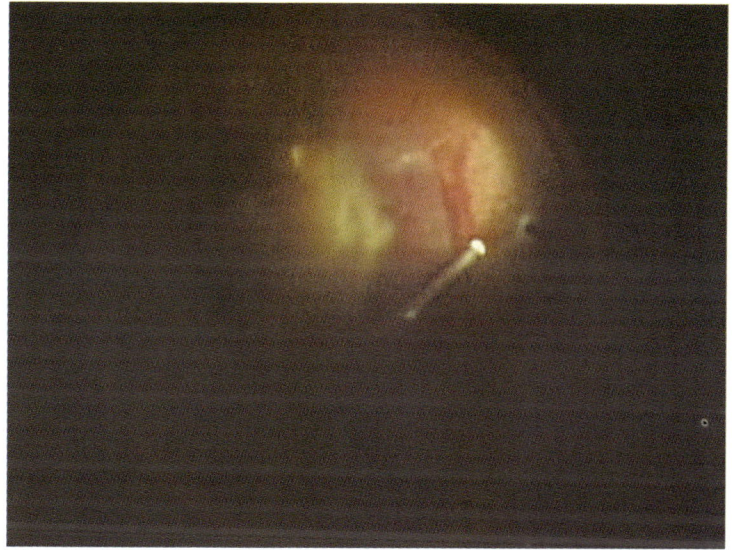

Fig. 5.3   Opening is extended toward the periphery.

Once an adequate potential space is created, the posterior hyaloid can be gently engaged by the cutter port, elevated and removed. Complete peripheral vitrectomy is then done.

The loose blood on the retina can then be removed using active or passive extrusion technique with a soft-tipped backflush needle/aspiration handpiece. Meticulous inspection of the retina is then done to look for any bleeders, which are then cauterized.

Once all the hemorrhage is removed and the bleeders cauterized, endolaser photocoagulation with either a sector or a complete panretinal photocoagulation is done.

Fluid-air exchange is done and the choice of tamponade is generally fluid or air unless there are chances of a rebleed, for which gas or silicone oil is a better option.

Special Points for Tractional Retinal Detachment

Apart from usual steps of surgery, in cases of TRD, PVD is usually absent and one should localize the traction points, which are potential sites for rhegmas and bleeders. After delineating such attachments, all new vessels are cauterized and the surrounding hyaloids are cut to prevent bleeding and countertraction to other areas of the retina, thus preventing break formation while removing the membranes.

Three types of traction relieving techniques have been described:

1. En bloc: This involves minimal core vitrectomy, traction release from beneath the hyaloid after creating an access to the retrohyaloid space, followed by en bloc removal of the vitreous. However, this is not the preferred technique.
2. Segmentation: This involves delineating attachments, segmenting bigger membranes into smaller ones to aid their removal (**Figs. 5.4A–D**).
3. Delamination: This involves release of traction point with peeling of the whole membrane (**Figs. 5.5A–C**).

Removal of fibrovascular tissue is best done with a combination of segmentation and delamination procedures where bridging areas of traction are divided and trimmed. The focal areas can be easily cut with a curved or horizontal or vertical scissors. After dividing and removing the focal attachments, the membranes can easily be peeled with an internal limiting membrane (ILM) forceps tangentially along the surface of the retina.

However, an added advantage in MIVS is that the port is closer to the tip of the cutter, allowing removal of epiretinal tissue by

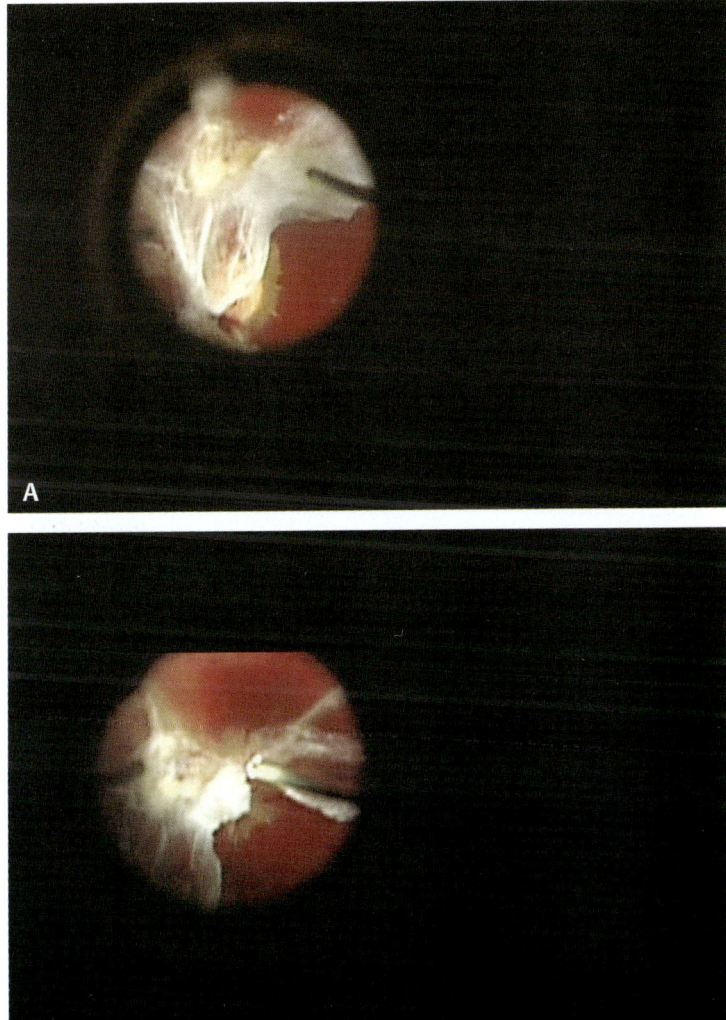

Fig. 5.4 **(A–B)** Technique of segmentation.

Contd.

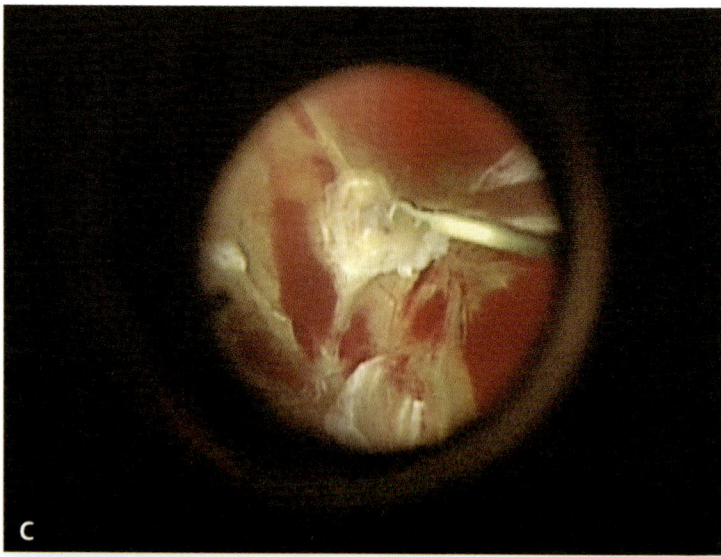

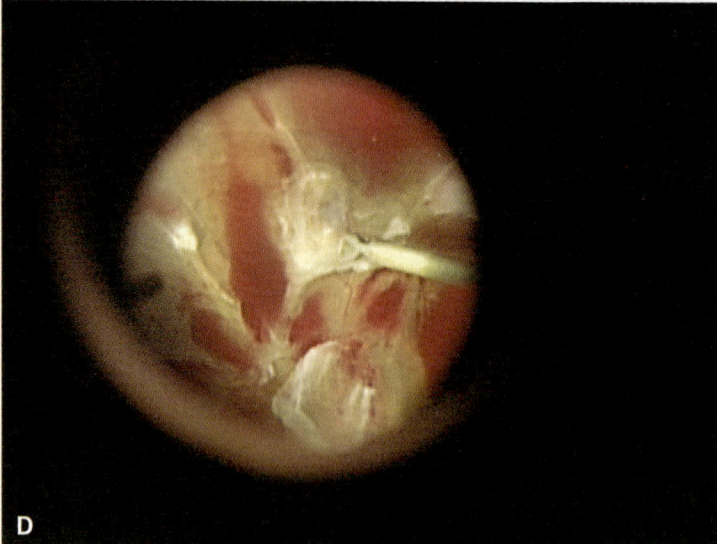

Fig. 5.4 **(C–D)** Technique of segmentation.

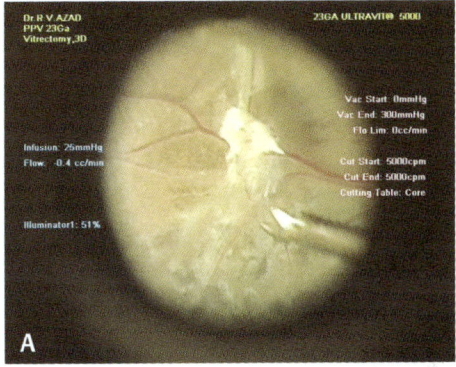

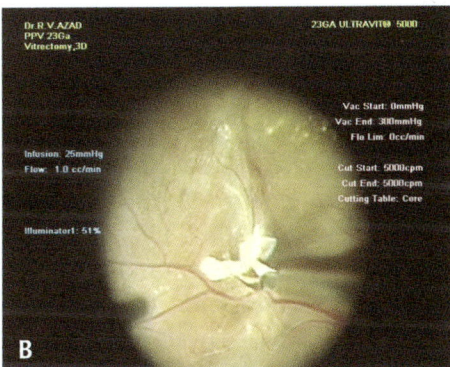

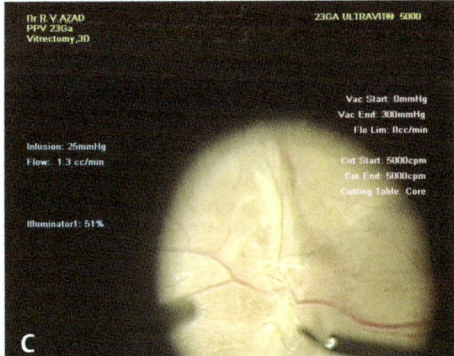

Fig. 5.5 **(A–C)** Delamination is being performed.

the cutter itself, especially in proliferative diabetic retinopathy. Hence, a cutter can perform all these steps too.

In the presence of firm adhesion of the proliferative tissue to the optic disc, traction should not be applied as this may cause bleeding; simply attachment to the disc can be trimmed by a vitreous cutter and left alone.

Bimanual surgery can also be attempted using a separate fourth port for the light, along with a scissors and forceps combination used to lift, peel, and expose the epicenters, offering precise control and avoiding iatrogenic retinal breaks.

Where the hyaloid is not easily identifiable, triamcinolone may be used to assist in the process for easy identification. Hyaloid should be removed completely to avoid redetachments.

Rarely one may encounter taut and thickened posterior hyaloid-like situation where no focal attachments can be delineated. Safer option for beginners is to leave the adherent hyaloid behind with meticulous panretinal photocoagulation and silicone oil injection and subsequent removal as a second-stage procedure when removal is easier, safer, and bloodless; or else, one may look for peripheral localized hyaloid detachment, which can be engaged and dissected centripetally rather than in the usual centrifugal pattern.

Intraoperative bleeding that may occur during dissection of fibrovascular membranes, especially when epicenters are cut, will also require aspiration and use of intraocular diathermy.

How to manage intraoperative bleeding?
1. Intraocular pressure is increased
2. Endodiathermy
3. Mechanical pressure with blunt instrument
4. Perfluorocarbon liquid
5. Fluid-air exchange
6. Port closure and wait

ILM peeling can be attempted as described in cases of recalcitrant macular edema.

These situations require a meticulous endolaser photocoagulation, and wide-angle viewing with the use of curved and extendable endolaser probes adds to our ability to achieve adequate ablation of the peripheral retina.

If traction is adequately removed and no iatrogenic or other retinal breaks are present and hemostasis is good, then no tamponade may be required. Alternatively, SF6 or C3F8 gas may be used where retinal breaks are present.

At the end of the procedure, a fluid–air exchange may be done for better sealing of the sclerotomies and to avoid postoperative hypotony.

Periphery screening especially in traumatic cases should be done for retinal breaks.

Indications of Oil

1. Intraoperative bleeding
2. Break formation with localized retinal detachment
3. Patients not maintaining positioning

Complications and Prognoses

The most important intra operative complication is profuse bleeding that may occur if adequate measures are not taken for prevention. Over zealous release of traction may lead to breaks and increase in the extent of RD making cases at times unsalvageable, so best avoided. Infusion pressures of more than 60 mm Hg should be kept for shortest required periods to avoid compromise to optic nerve head perfusion. Late rebleed can also occur. Prognoses largely depends on macular and optic nerve head status and recovery may take longer than usual.

Surgical Tips

- ✓ Preoperative work-up, ultrasonography, anti-VEGF, and laser
- ✓ Prognostication, systemic optimization, other eye management
- ✓ Proper assessment of PVD/RD before making an opening
- ✓ Careful retrohyaloid aspiration of blood for better visualization of retina
- ✓ Cautery, segmentation, delamination, and managing bleeders

Rhegmato-genous Retinal Detachment

Shorya Vardhan Azad and Brijesh Takkar

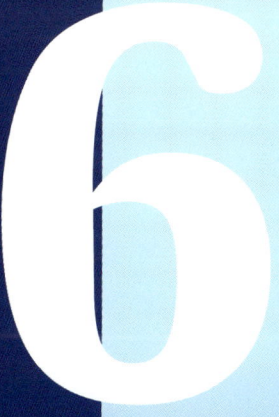

6

6 Rhegmatogenous Retinal Detachment

Introduction

In its early stages of development, indications of vitreous surgery for repair of retinal detachments were limited to complex cases. However, pars plana vitrectomy is now being used as primary procedure in certain uncomplicated retinal detachments as well. By direct removal of vitreous bands, vitreoretinal tractional membranes, and subretinal membranes, vitrectomy allows nearly total elimination of vitreous traction. It creates space for injection of vitreous substitutes such as long-acting gases and silicone oil. Simultaneous scleral buckling can also be done.

Preoperative Assessment

Systemic history should be taken and all efforts should be made to rule out cases of exudative retinal detachment and secondary rhegmatogenous retinal detachment (RRD). Duration of symptoms guides us toward prognosis of the detachment and the timing of surgery. Some detachments with proliferative vitreoretinopathy (PVR) which have immature membranes can be delayed till the membranes mature, aiding in their easier removal. Visual assessment is very important as it is a guide toward functional prognosis. Projection of rays (PR) should be checked properly, and inaccurate PR in absence of giant retinal tear, dense media opacities, and endophthalmitis should be alarming. Anterior segment examination should be done carefully in cases of trauma and also where associated cataract might be present. Significant cataract may require combined surgery or pars plana lensectomy. In cases where there are media opacities, ultrasonography should be performed to look for retinal detachment with special importance to the mobility and configuration (funnel) of the detachment, as it might change our management. A meticulous examination of retina should be performed with indirect ophthalmoscopy, noting extent, all breaks, macular status, posterior vitreous detachment (PVD), and amount of PVR. Depending on the complexity of RD, patient should be counseled about surgery and its realistic outcomes. Hypotony is usually present with RRD, but intraocular pressure (IOP) may be high in Schwartz syndrome or traumatic RRD. In severe hypotony with choroidal detachment (CD), a short course of steroids can be prescribed to build up the IOP before posting for elective surgery. Neovascularization of iris, chronic uveitis, chronic CD, and anterior PVR are indicators of longstanding RRD.

Fellow eye management should be done as required. Scleral buckling may be combined depending on surgeon preference.

Surgery

Choice of vitreous surgery versus primary scleral buckling depends on the surgeon preference. Three-port vitrectomy is done (20/23/25-gauge) as already discussed earlier.

In the presence of CD, one should opt for 6-mm cannula or change the location of the cannula away from the CD. The location of the cannula tip should always be confirmed before switching on the infusion.

Sclerotomy sites should be devoid of the vitreous to prevent port-site complications.

Initially, core vitrectomy is done to remove bulk of the central vitreous gel. Cut rate of 3,500 cpm and suction pressure of 300 to 350 mm Hg are sufficient in 23 gauge. Extensive core vitrectomy should be avoided as it hampers easy gripping of the hyaloids for PVD induction.

Staining of the posterior hyaloid with steroid is advisable for the beginners as the edge of the hyaloid becomes more apparent (**Fig. 6.1**). Posterior hyaloid is then separated from the retinal surface by applying active suction over the optic disc with the cutter/soft-tipped cannula. Generally, suction pressure of around 250 to 350 mm Hg (depending of gauge) is enough, although younger patients, especially pediatric age group, might need higher suction pressure for PVD induction. One should remember to increase the IOP at this time to counter the higher suction pressure.

After PVD induction, one should shift to wide-angle viewing system and the hyaloid is lifted as anteriorly as possible and peripheral vitrectomy is completed. In cases of difficult induction, surgeon may use soft-tipped cannula passively or forceps to loosen the edges (**Fig. 6.1**).

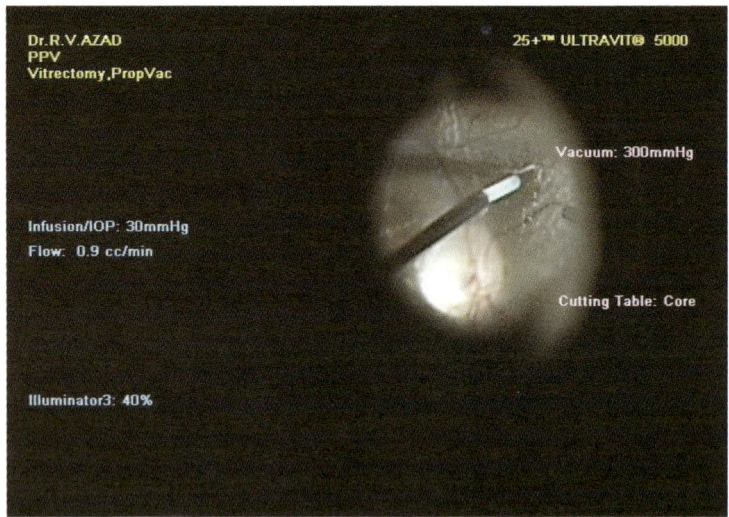

Fig. 6.1 Triamcinolone stained hyaloid being loosened with soft tip.

Anterior traction on the break is relieved by suction and shaving the vitreous base as much as possible with the cutter (**Figs. 6.2** and **6.3**). During peripheral vitrectomy, the cut rate should be maximum and suction pressure should be reduced to 50 to 200 mm Hg (depending of gauge) to avoid traction on peripheral retina and iatrogenic break formation (**Fig. 6.4**). Anterior flaps of horseshoe tears should always be removed. In phakic patients, scleral indentation should be done to complete vitrectomy. Although not always possible, one should aim for complete vitreous removal, which includes both cortical and medullary vitreous. This is the best time to manage PVR as discussed ahead.

Subretinal fluid (SRF) is drained either through preexisting retinal breaks or through creation of a drainage retinotomy. Internal drainage can be done passively with backflush or actively with soft-tipped cannula (**Fig. 6.5**). Posterior retinotomy is created

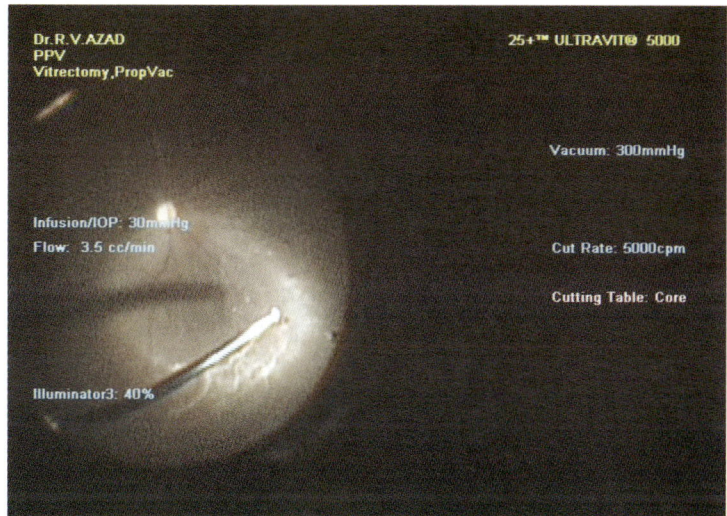

Fig. 6.2 Relieving vitreous traction over the break.

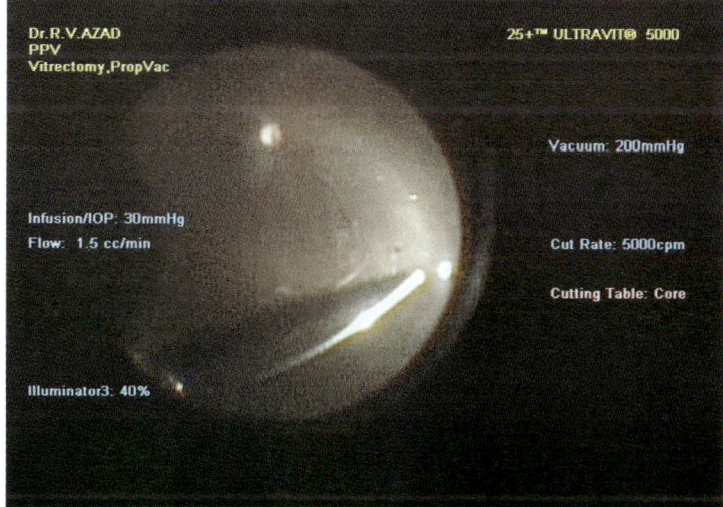

Fig. 6.3 Vitreous base dissection.

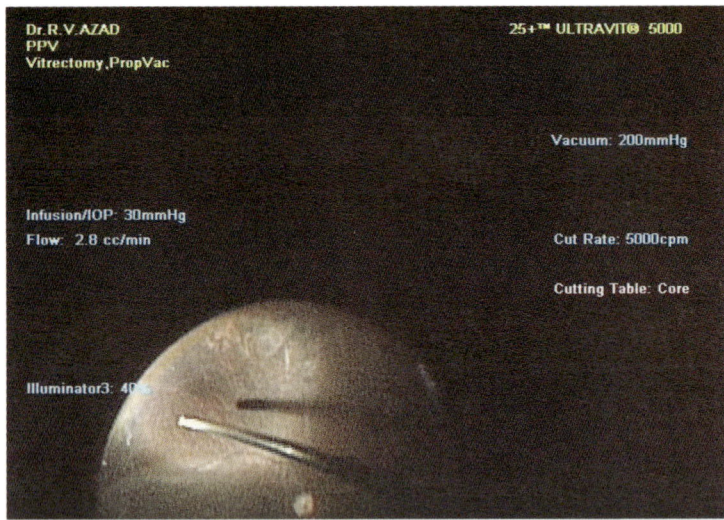

Fig. 6.4 Peripheral vitrectomy.

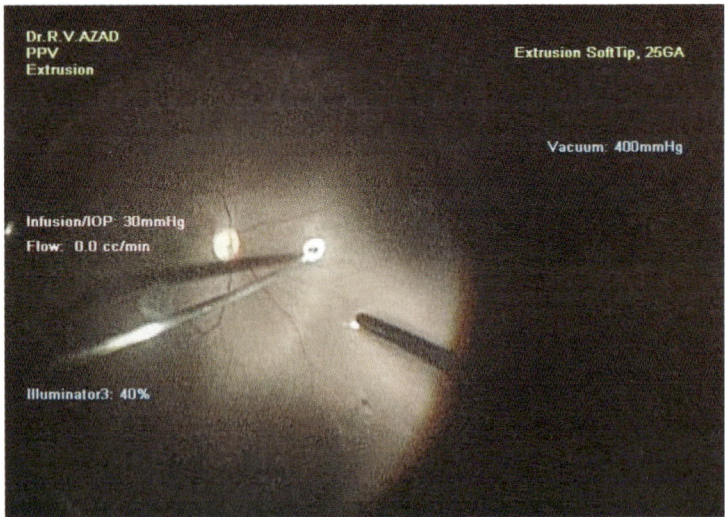

Fig. 6.5 Internal drainage with soft tipped cannula through posterior retinotomy.

generally in an avascular area superonasal to the disc with the help of electric cautery. The instrument of choice is placed at the retinotomy site and fluid–air exchange (FAX) is initiated. SRF is drained and FAX is completed. Once retina is attached, retinopexy is done with laser/cryotherapy. Posterior retinal breaks are treated with laser photocoagulation using endolaser probe (**Figs. 6.6–6.8**). Anterior breaks not amenable to laser retinopexy can be sealed with the help of cryotherapy.

Perfluorocarbon liquids (PFCLs) are heavier than water and are being increasingly used temporarily during the surgery. They help in steam rolling of posteriorly pooled SRF to anteriorly placed retinotomies or breaks.

Before lasering around the posterior retinotomy, a soft-tipped cannula should be used to drain the residual SRF. Inability to

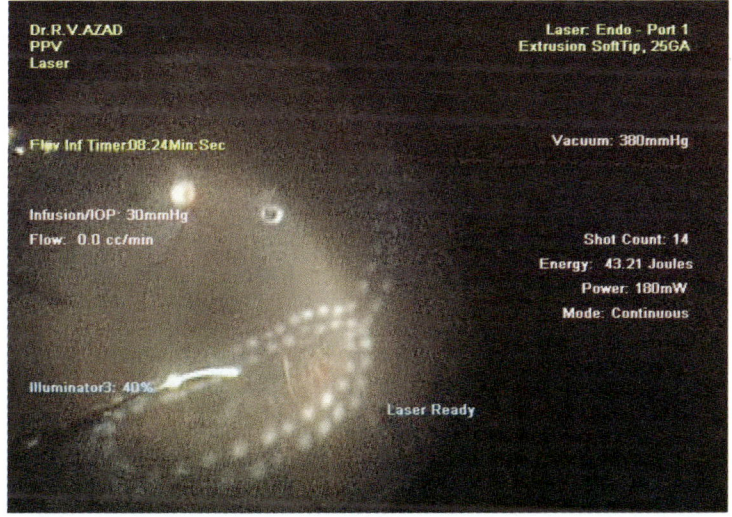

Fig. 6.6 Laser photocoagulation around the break and lattice degeneration.

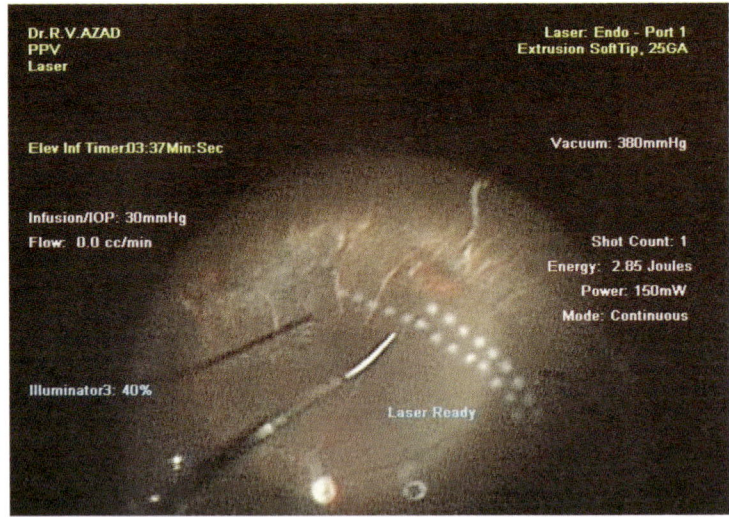

Fig. 6.7 360-degree Laser photocoagulation.

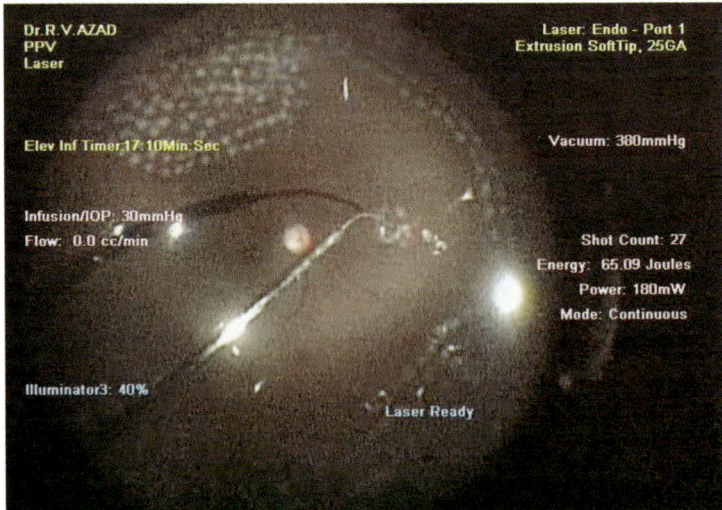

Fig. 6.8 Laser photocoagulation around the posterior retinotomy.

attain adequate greyish-white burns indicates residual SRF, retinal edema, traction, dehydrated retina, or retinal pigment epithelium (RPE) dropout (myopes).

Depending upon the location of breaks, number of breaks, and additional pathology, internal tamponade is done by using short-acting agents, such as sulfur hexafluoride (SF6), or long-acting agents, such as perfluoropropane (C3F8) or silicone oil. Silicone oil is removed after 3 to 6 months.

Special Techniques for PVR (Epiretinal/ Subretinal/Intraretinal)

Scleral buckle elements such as segmental buckles, circumferential buckle and encircling bands may be used additionally depending upon the need for traction relief. The surgeon may also anticipate post-op PVR (pediatric/traumatic/CD/inferior breaks) and opt for such a support.

The buckle relieves the anteroposterior traction and closes peripheral breaks. It also relieves circumferential retinal traction. The posterior retina gets a more posterior "ora Serrata" at the posterior edge of the buckle. Prophylactic band may be applied where inadequate vitrectomy is expected (lattices/myope/phakic/media opacities).

If the view is obscured by cataract, the lens should be removed and anterior capsular rim can be left for future IOL implantation. However, with the advent of wide-angle viewing system, requirement of removal of lens has been reduced to a great extent.

A meticulous pars plana vitrectomy is performed and complete vitrectomy done in anterior PVR. Removal of anterior traction is done with the help of wide-angle viewing systems, and scleral depression may also be used for visualization of the vitreous base. Elective lensectomy may be needed.

The posterior membranes can be identified with the help of the light pipe by varying the obliqueness and using vitreoretinal pick to elevate the edge of the membrane. A membrane pic forceps, particularly, is useful for this purpose as it can help elevate the membrane in the closed position and then can be used to grasp and carefully strip the membrane (**Figs. 6.9** and **6.10**).

With the advent of xenon and metal halide illumination systems, a trocar cannula chandelier of 25 gauge can be used at a convenient location so as to accomplish bimanual dissection of membrane.

The anterior vitreoretinal proliferations (anterior PVR) are tightly attached and require a combination of scissor dissection and forceps to remove them: particularly from the vitreous base, the bimanual technique is surgically safer and more effective for proliferation in the anterior area. PFCL can be used to stabilize the posterior retina and as a third hand. If unsuccessful, triamcinolone-assisted removal with forceps, diamond-dusted membrane scraper, or soft-tip cannula can be attempted.

If subretinal fibrotic bands exist as subretinal dendritic strands or as an annular ring near the optic disc (napkin ring) and are causing traction, they need to be removed. This can be done via existing breaks or by creating a small retinotomy. Subretinal forceps can be used to grasp and remove those proliferations, which are normally not as adherent. End-gripping forceps are best and can be rotated to "noodle out" (**Figs. 6.11–6.16**) the subretinal bands in a traction-free manner. Peripheral sub-retinal band (SRB) with no posterior extensions can be best left alone.

Once all traction is relieved, FAX with drainage of SRF is done through either an existing break or a retinotomy using a soft-tipped backflush needle.

Anchoring 360-degree laser is beneficial as pre-op PVR is an indicator of post-op PVR. The final buckle tie are then tightened and a reasonably high buckle indent is achieved in the air-filled eye.

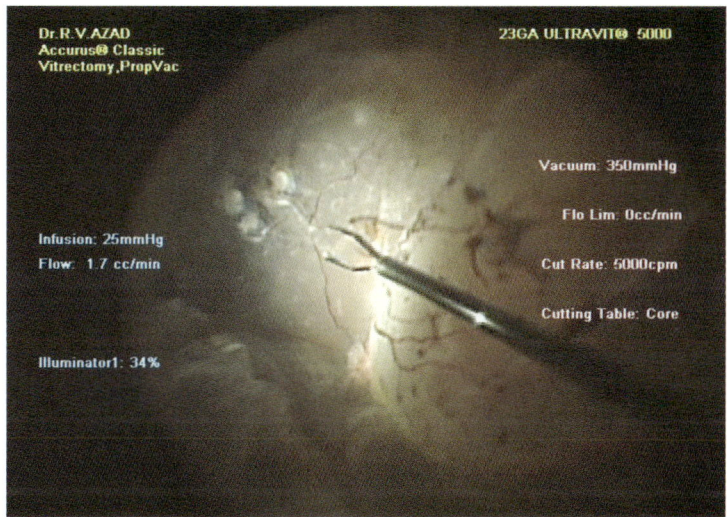

Fig. 6.9 Membrane being gripped with forceps.

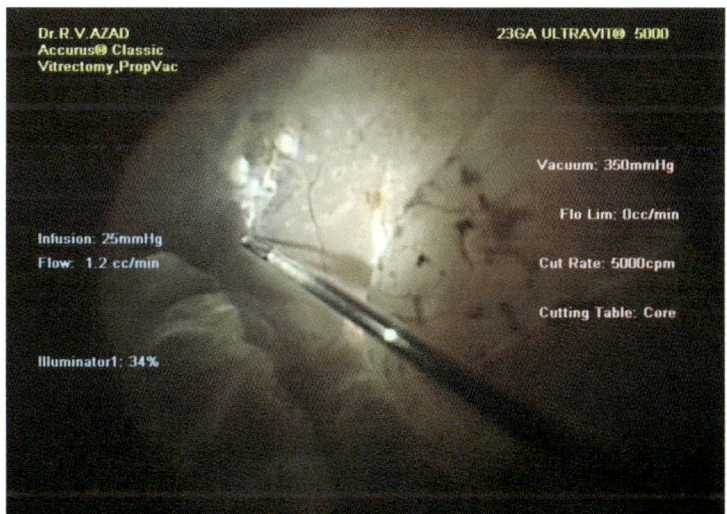

Fig. 6.10 Membrane separated from the retina.

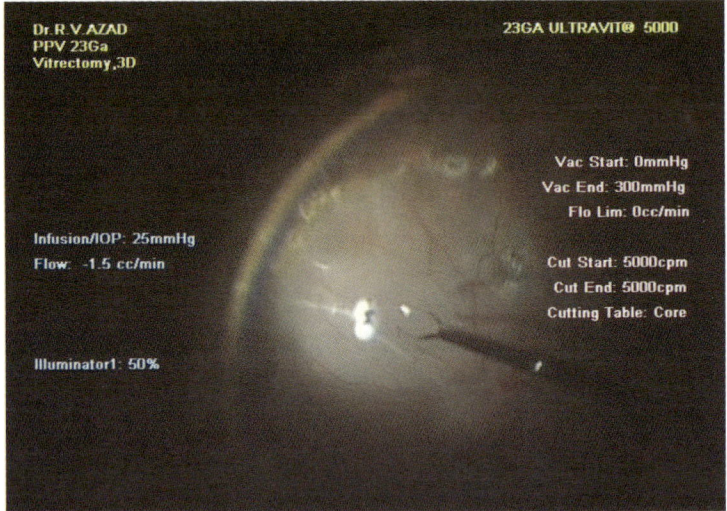

Fig. 6.11 Retinotomy made adjacent to the subretinal band.

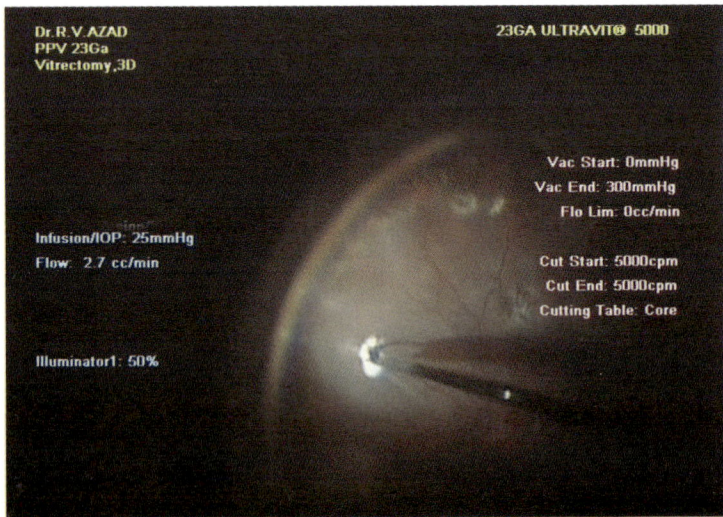

Fig. 6.12 The subretinal band grasped through the retinotomy with forceps.

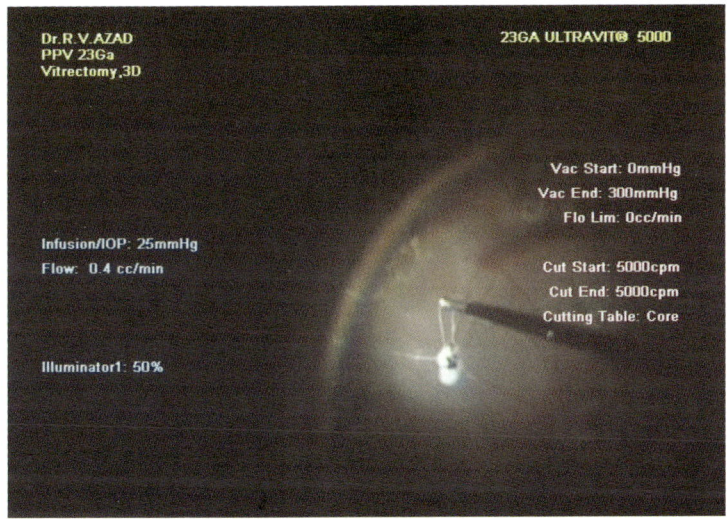

Fig. 6.13 The subretinal band noodled out in vitreous cavity.

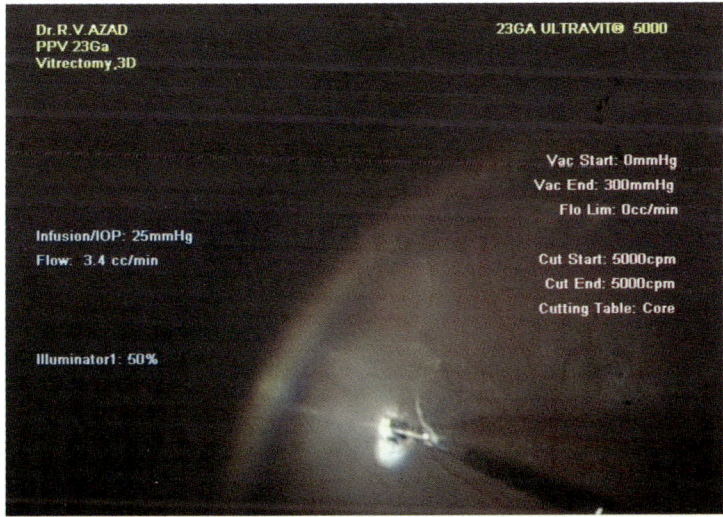

Fig. 6.14 One end of the subretinal band prolapsed into the vitreous cavity.

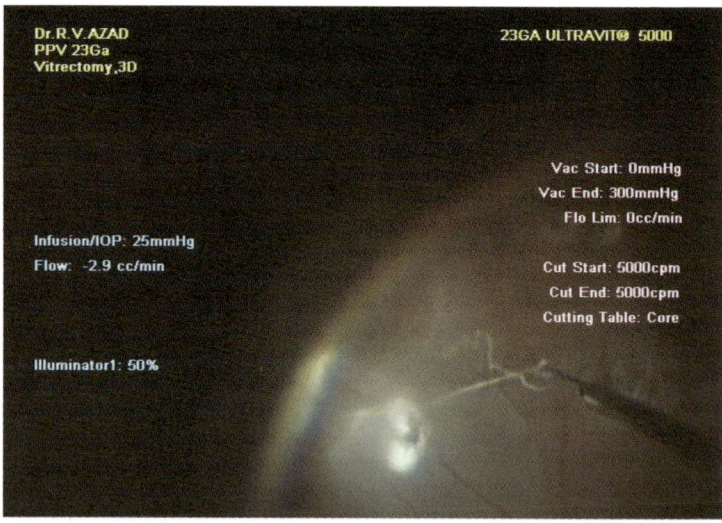

Fig. 6.15 Remaining subretinal portion of the band being externalized.

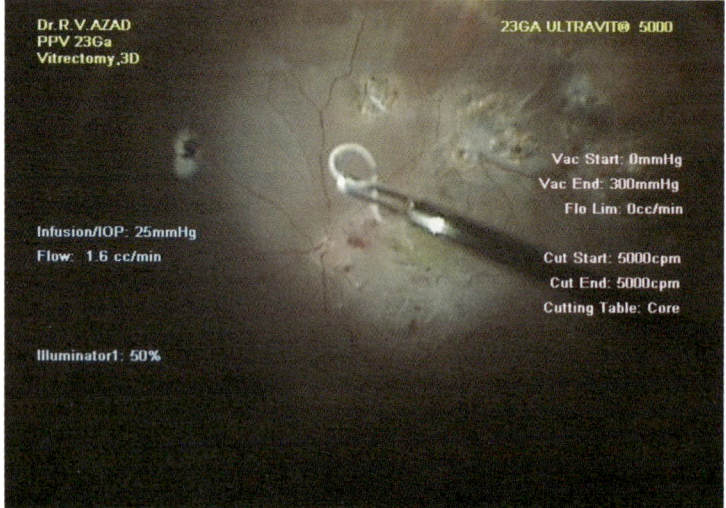

Fig. 6.16 Successful removal of the subretinal band.

If on endodrainage and an adequate buckle height, retina is not opposed to RPE, air may enter subretinal space (refer to Chapter 13, Fig. 13.3). It indicates unrelieved traction, intraretinal PVR, and/or high indent. A decision on additional relaxing retinotomy and retinectomy has to be taken now and this should only be done once all membranes have been adequately removed.

For retinectomies, PFCL should be injected (**Fig. 6.17**) before to prevent submacular migration of possible bleed. Size of relaxing retinectomies is best judged under air, but is far easier and safer under fluid after diathermy of the proposed area as bleeding is much easier to manage (**Figs. 6.18–6.20**). The edges of the retinectomy should be oriented radially pointing toward the ora.

These relaxing retinotomies or retinectomies are performed in presence of retinal incarcerations in traumatic or surgical wounds, fibrous proliferations, and severe intrinsic retinal contractions. The peripheral retina is sacrificed in these retinectomies to protect the functionally important posterior retina. At times, just radial peripheral relaxing retinotomies (**Figs. 6.21–6.23**) may be enough to relieve circumferential contraction and avoid 360-degree retinectomy.

Although our aim is to remove all possible PVR (epi/sub), at times we can remove the residual PVR at the time of silicone oil removal (SOR) or even as a planned second surgery. Overzealous removal of PVR can actually lead to complications, making the case unsalvageable, and hence best avoided.

Last but not the least is the choice of suitable tamponade; both silicone oil and a nonexpansile mixture of perfluoropropane gas can be used as both have advantages and disadvantages. As a general rule, we like 14 to 15% C3F8 gas, where less PVR is present and a shorter duration tamponade is necessary (3–4 weeks). In cases requiring extensive surgery, that is, in advanced case of PVR where a few months of retinal stabilization are needed, silicone oil (1,000–5,000 cSt) is the proven choice.

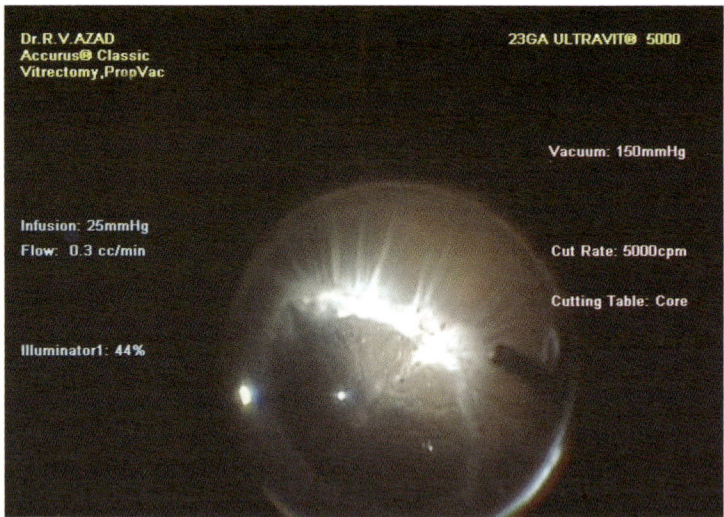

Fig. 6.17 Severe anterior proliferative vitreoretinopathy preventing flattening of retina despite perfluorocarbon liquids.

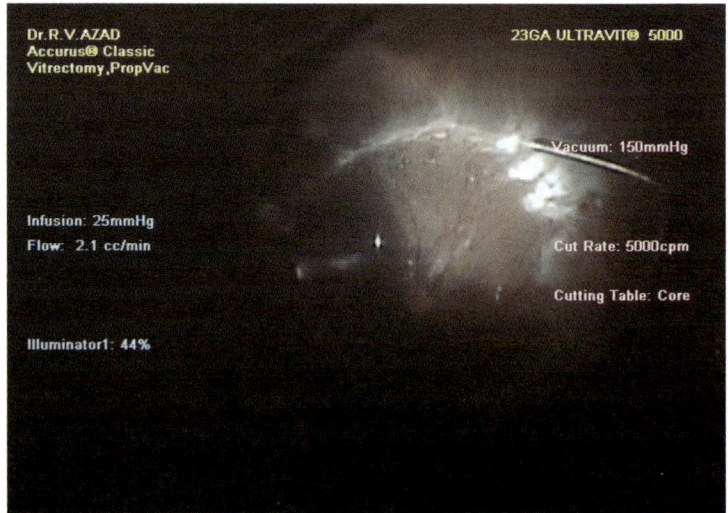

Fig. 6.18 Diathermy at the planned site of relaxing retinectomy.

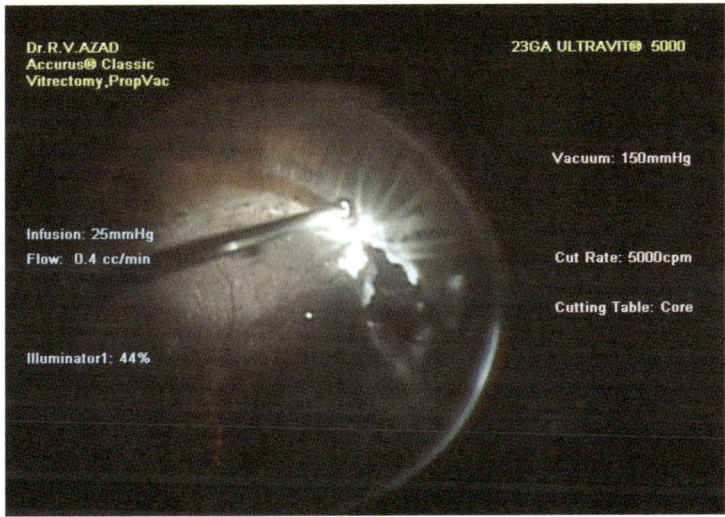

Fig. 6.19 Retinectomy being performed with cutter.

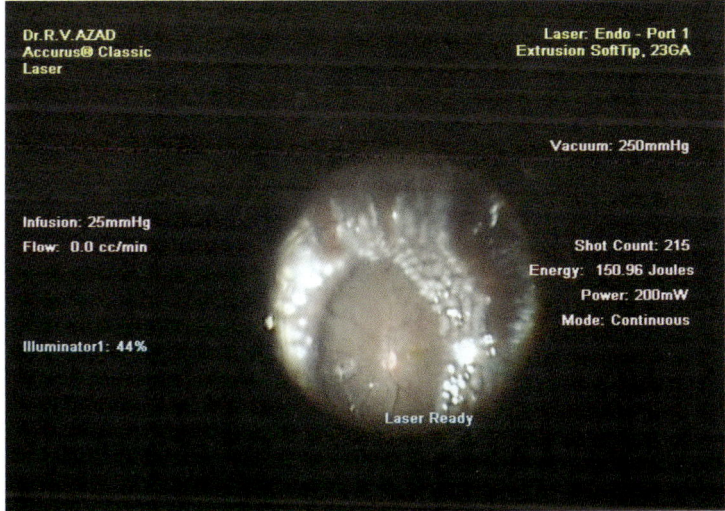

Fig. 6.20 Retina settled and lasered under air.

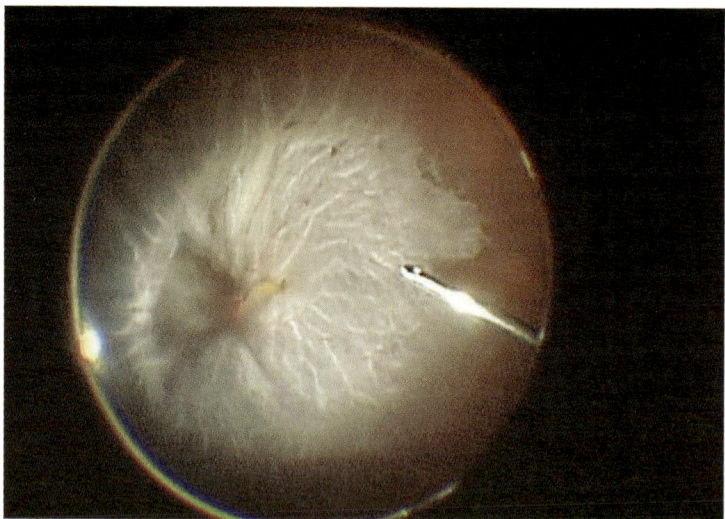

Fig. 6.21 Severe circumferential retinal shortening.

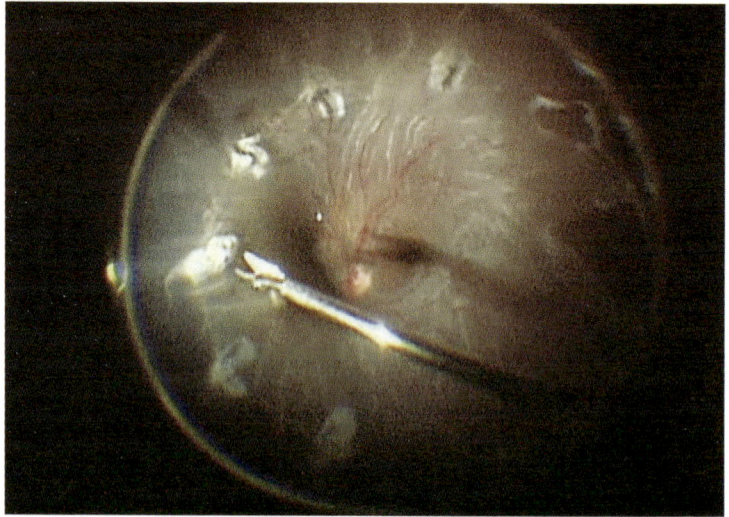

Fig. 6.22 Multiple relaxing retinotomies being made with scissors.

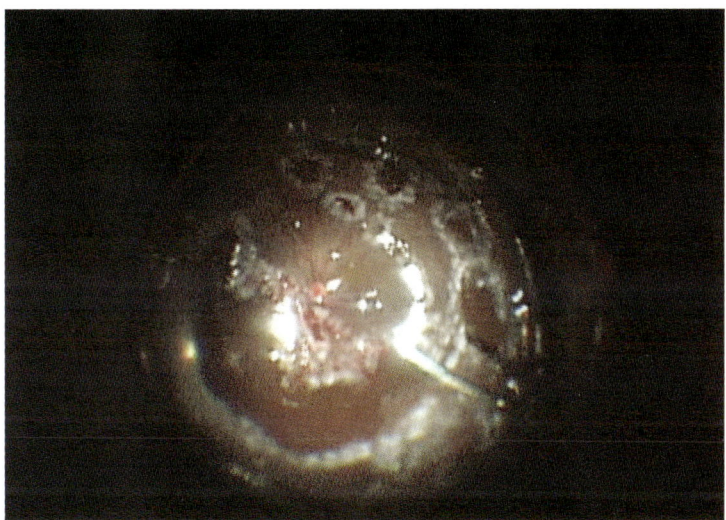

Fig. 6.23 Retina settled and lasered under air.

In patients with more complex RRD, primary pars plana vitrectomy is done more frequently with fewer complications. The precise role of primary pars plana vitrectomy in new uncomplicated retinal detachment remains debatable owing to the lack of controlled randomized trials. PVR surgery remains a challenging surgery even for the experienced surgeon as the course of the PVR may progress even after successful repair.

Complications and Prognoses

Complications during surgery for retinal detachment, may vary and are described in detail in Chapter 13. Functional prognosis depends on the duration of RD, macular/optic disc status and is the best for macula on RDs. Advanced PVR and intraretinal short-ening may make cases inoperable. Postoperatively, redetach-ments may occur despite initial anatomical success, especially in cases with pre-op PVR, inadequate retinopexy and poor tampon-ading effect.

Surgical Tips

✓ Prudent case selection and preoperative judge-ment of final visual outcome

✓ Patient counseling in high risk cases

✓ Decision for encirclage

✓ Adequate vitrectomy and careful PVD induction

✓ Manage PVR removing all visible traction

✓ Slow internal drainage

✓ Correct choice of tamponading agent

✓ Post operative patient positioning

Giant Retinal Tear

Brijesh Takkar and Shorya Vardhan Azad

7

7 Giant Retinal Tear

Introduction

Giant retinal tear (GRT) is much more than just a large retinal tear. Defined as a full-thickness retinal break extending beyond 90 degrees, its varied clinical presentations, fellow eye management, proliferative vitreoretinopathy (PVR), and difficult surgery make GRT a different entity. Initially, a GRT retinal detachment (RD) had a very poor prognosis, but introduction of perfluorocarbon liquids (PFCLs) later has improved the results and also simplified the difficult surgical steps.

Preoperative Assessment

Idiopathic GRTs constitute more than half of the cases, while the rest are myopic, traumatic, iatrogenic, or syndromic such as Marfan, Stickler, and Ehler–Danlos. Apart from trauma, its pathogenesis involves initial central vitreous liquefaction and peripheral condensation along the vitreous base, which, on contraction, allows for formation of large breaks in a zipper fashion in the peripheral retina. Often, radial horns are present at the edge of the GRT, and rupture of the retinal vessels causes vitreous hemorrhage. Therefore, posterior vitreous detachment (PVD) is generally present apart from traumatic cases. Also, the large area of bare choroid allows for dispersion of retinal pigment epithelium cells and fulminant PVR in quick time, requiring timely surgery.

Projection of light may be inaccurate due to the large disruption in function, and does not necessarily mean poor prognoses. Hypotony and choroidal detachment may be present with inflammation. Preoperative steroids hence would make surgery easier. PVR is present in late-presenting cases and evaluation in total GRTs is very difficult as the whole retina lies crumpled up posteriorly. Macular holes and more tears may be present. Lens status should be considered specifically as clear lens lensectomies may be needed.

Giant Tear versus Dialysis

Traumatic GRTs may not have a PVD. Also, trauma can cause dialysis rather than a tear. They can be differentiated by absence of radial extensions, absence of PVD, less PVR, and slow progression of RD in GRD as compared to GRT. The biggest difference, however, lies in the fact that while vitreous base is attached to the anterior flap of the GRT, it is attached to the posterior edge of the dialysis, thus allowing for rolling of the posterior retinal flap in GRT and not in GRD. This posterior flap in essence is what makes the surgery in GRT an altogether different entity and its management is extremely essential for successful reattachment of retina. A giant dialysis may be associated with vitreous base avulsion.

Giant tears should be treated as emergency, as they become unmanageable with severe PVR very soon.

Surgery

- A GRT detected early before the development of RD can be treated with laser photocoagulation only.

- *Role of encirclage*: This remains a controversy, as, despite numerous reports confirming equally successful management without explants, many surgeons continue to use it. Point in favor is the support provided to the vitreous base especially at sites away from the tear and against being the risk of retinal slippage. Perhaps, it is safest to use explants in the presence of inferior PVR, GRD, or additional inferior breaks. Shallow indent should be given if encirclage is planned.

- *Managing the lens*: Cataractous lens requires lensectomy. Although wide-angle viewing systems have simplified anterior and vitreous base management, phakic cases still may present with difficulty. It is better to perform a lensectomy rather than compromising vitrectomy even in clear lens cases. Intraocular lens may be explanted if subluxated, and often poor management of cataract surgery is the cause of GRT in the first place.

- *Vitrectomy*: Inserting the infusion cannula in hypotonous eyes requires patience. If the cannula is found to be subchoroidal in the already inflamed eye, one can insert a

89

second instrument such as an MVR from opposite port to clear the loose choroidal tissue from the cannula opening. Alternatively, a fresh site or a 6-mm cannula may be used in 20-gauge surgeries. A radical dissection of the vitreous base should be performed using modern instrumentation (**Fig. 7.1**). Edges of the GRT should be freshened especially in the presence of PVR and contracture.

- *Anterior retinal flap*: It should be removed as it is functionally redundant and if left can fibrose and can either pull the ciliary body or develop PVR at the edges to cause recurrent detachment.

- *PVR*: Standard management is required. In special situations, the GRT may be extended (sometimes 360 degrees) till the peripheral traction is relieved.

- *PFCL injection*: Due to its high specific gravity, low viscosity, different refractive index, and transparency, PFCL is a great advantage in inverting the rolled-up flap of GRT (**Fig. 7.2**). One should, however, release the posterior PVR before injecting the same as otherwise it may go subretinal. PFCL should be injected till it reaches the edge of the GRT (**Fig. 7.3**). In severe retinal contracture, the retina may not flatten even at the posterior pole and one may have to abandon such a surgery.

- *Retinopexy*: Laser photocoagulation is then done with at least four to five rows around the GRT and its edge. It is advisable to do a 360-degree endolaser (**Fig. 7.4A, B**). As the peripheral retina can still have pockets of fluid, it may not readily take up laser reaction and may require laser after the oil exchange.

- *PFCL–air exchange*: It is important to keep the edge of the GRT dry. Hence, a slow exchange should be attempted,

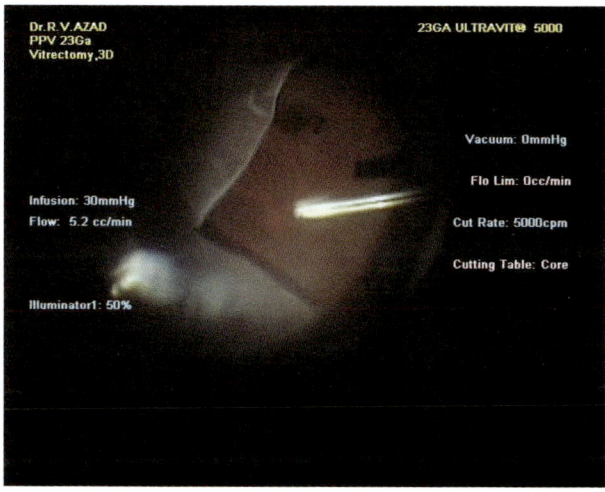

Fig. 7.1 Radical vitreous base dissection being done over giant retinal tear.

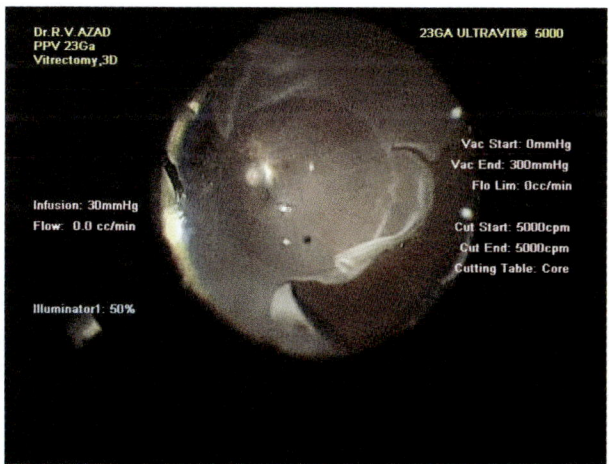

Fig. 7.2 Unrolling of giant retinal tear flap with perfluorocarbon liquids.

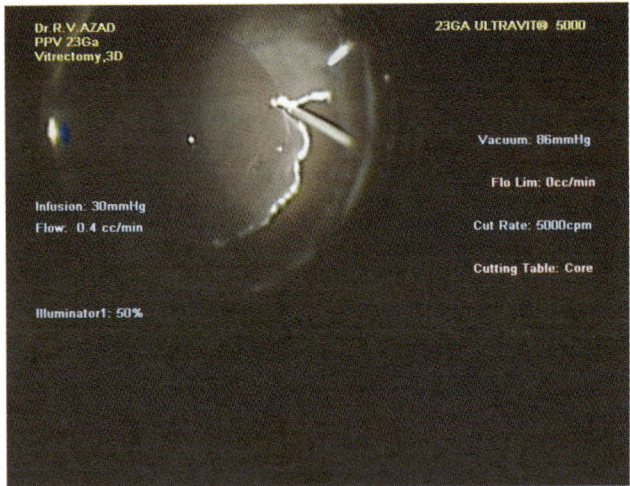

Fig. 7.3 Perfluorocarbon liquids injected till the posterior cauterized edge of giant retinal tear.

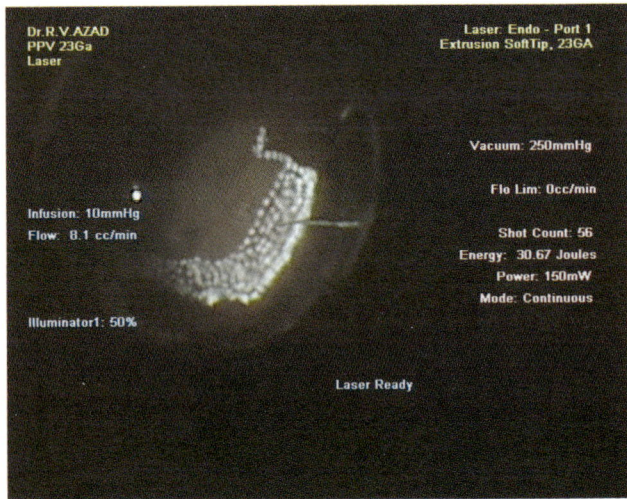

Fig. 7.4(A) Four to five rows of Laser at the edge of giant retinal tear.

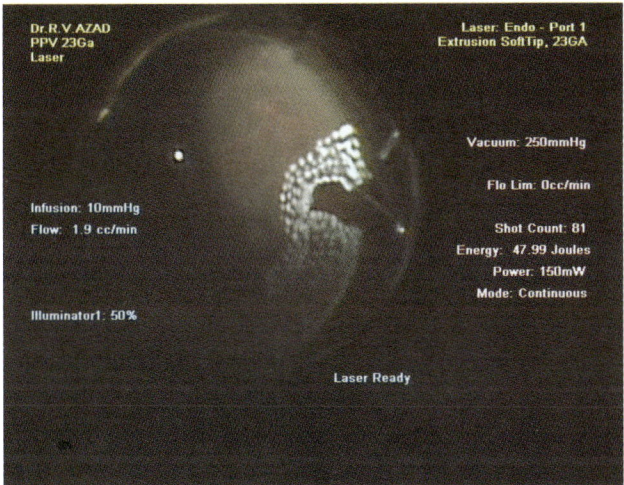

Fig. 7.4(B) Four to five rows of Laser at the edge of giant retinal tear.

which should be interrupted again and again if retinal folds are seen. Such folds indicate retinal slippage. A patiently done PFCL–air exchange with soft-tipped cannula/gentle extrusion does not cause problems.

- *PFCL–oil exchange*: This has the least chances of retinal slippage but may be difficult for a novice surgeon. The difficulty lies in managing the pockets of peripheral fluid left and the fluid that starts accumulating between the PFCL and the oil once the exchange is initialized. To achieve this, the suction instrument should be placed just underneath the PFCL bubble and one should keep lowering the instrument as the exchange progresses (**Fig. 7.5**). Intermittently, one can go to the retinal edge to ensure it is dry, as mentioned earlier. The small bore of the suction device can get clogged by the oil, leading to high intraocular pressure, and early detection of clogging is advisable.

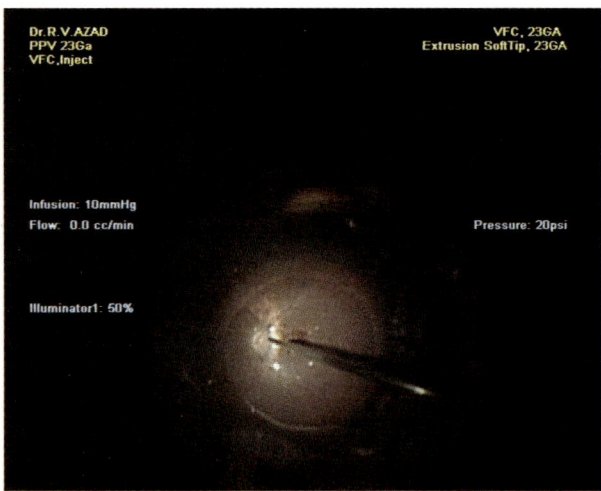

Fig. 7.5 Perfluorocarbon liquid-oil exchange.

- Heavy oils are a new inclusion but still more experience is needed with them. One may leave PFCL for a week or so and perform the exchange as a second procedure. Associated macular holes, cataract, and other pathologies require management accordingly.

Complications and Prognoses

In the modern era, the surgical results in GRT have greatly improved. Oil is generally preferred over gas, although equal results have been reported in the literature. Good visual acuity and anatomical results can be achieved if early surgery is performed in the absence of pre-op PVR. Subretinal bleed, subretinal/retained PFCL, retinal folds, and hyphema are known to be associated with cleanest of surgeries. Post-op PVR remains a difficult area due to bare choroid and cell dispersion and can lead to recurrent RD.

Surgical Tips

- ✓ Complete vitrectomy and vitreous base shaving
- ✓ PFCL and wide-angle viewing systems
- ✓ During PFCL exchange, retinal edge to be kept dry and PFCL to be completely removed
- ✓ Managing lens and 4-5 rows of laser

Macular Surgeries

Brijesh Takkar and Shorya Vardhan Azad

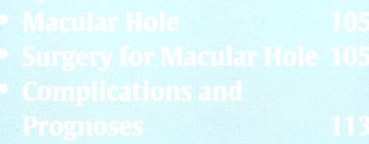
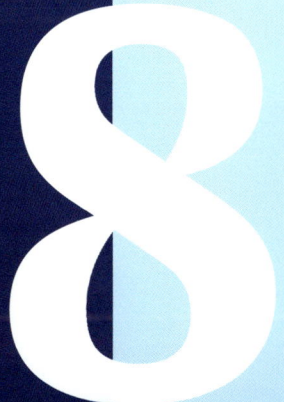

8

8 Macular Surgeries

Introduction

From the days when macular surgeries were virtually unknown, we have now come to an era of ophthalmic surgery where macular surgeries perhaps have the best visual prognoses. Better understanding of the pathogenesis of epiretinal membranes (ERMs) and macular holes (MHs) has changed the surgical approach. Other indications include vitreomacular traction (VMT), cystoid macular edema (CME), age-related macular degeneration, and subretinal bleeds.

Preoperative Assessment

A complete history of macular symptoms, such as metamorphopsia and scotoma, and their duration should be asked as leading questions. History of trauma/prior ocular procedures should always be acquired because of obvious functional and anatomical implications. Best corrected visual acuity (BCVA) should always be sought, and patients with BCVA better than 6/12 should not be operated on unless they are visually very disturbed due to metamorphopsia or due to professional requirements. Poor presenting visual acuity indicates chronicity as well as severity of the disease. Similarly, those with BCVA below 4/60 should be thoroughly evaluated for other causes of vision loss. Apart from the regular work-up, presence of posterior subcapsular cataract and media disturbing cortical cataract should alert the surgeon to the possible requirement for cataract surgery before vitrectomy. ERMs and MHs are very commonly associated with peripheral tears, and such findings should always be searched for. Grading of ERM/MH should be done for better prognostication. Posterior vitreous detachment (PVD) is usually present in idiopathic ERM and stage 4 MH. Optical coherence tomography (OCT) has led to a better understanding and management of macular cases, and is therefore a must for these cases.

Epiretinal Membrane

ERMs can be broadly divided as idiopathic, secondary (retinal vein occlusion, uveitis, trauma, etc.), and iatrogenic (cataract, laser, etc.). While grade 0 ERMs constitute the majority and can be followed up, grades 1 and 2 may require surgical management. Examination and OCT may elucidate pseudo/true MH, which may require management accordingly. Foveal contour also determines outcomes.

Surgery for Epiretinal Membrane

Careful case selection and informed consent should be obtained. Visual recovery after ERM surgery occurs over long periods ranging from months to years.

- *Microinvasive vitrectomy system* is the preferred vitrectomy system. Standard pars plana vitrectomy (PPV) is done.

- *Triamcinolone* is injected to visualize hyaloid (**Fig. 8.1**). It is important to stain over the disc as well as macula. Gentle induction should be done to avoid macular breaks that may occur in strongly adherent ERMs. Steroid crystals rest on the hyaloid, allowing for easier and safer PVD induction.

- *Active suction* with the cutter itself or soft-tipped cannula may be done. Bending of the cannula on engagement of hyaloids has been described as the "fish strike sign." Pick forceps, bent micro vitreo-retinal (MVR) knife, and membrane forceps may be used when necessary.

- *Peripheral vitrectomy* is completed.

- *Staining the ERM.* Various dyes are available. Currently, trypan blue may be used to stain the ERM, or brilliant blue green (BBG) may be used for negative staining. Both are safe, especially in the absence of MH.

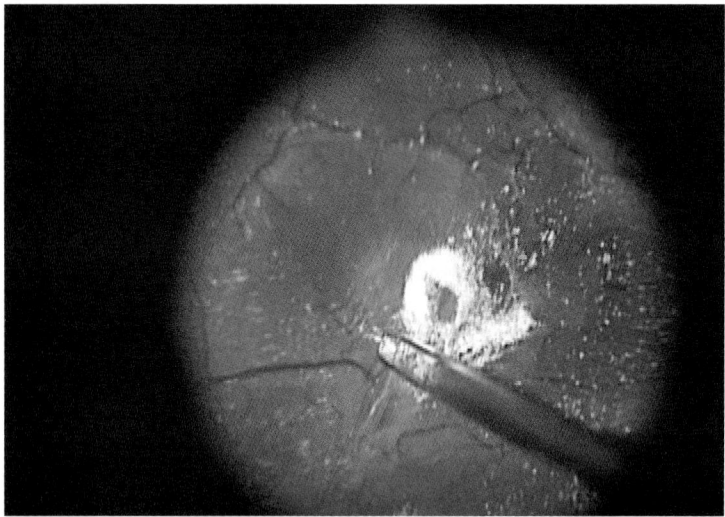

Fig. 8.1 Edge of the membrane grasped after staining with triamcinolone.

- *Engaging and peeling ERMs*: If a thick edge is available (**Fig. 8.1**), forceps may be used directly to gently peel the stained ERM. Alternatively, bent MVR, diamond-dusted membrane scraper (DDMS), and pick forceps may be used to create an edge. A skilled surgeon may directly impinge the ERM with forceps and apply "tangential" traction (**Figs. 8.2** and **8.3**). The surgeon should be attentive to avoid retinal damage while applying traction. If an adherent area in ERM is encountered, the ERM should be approached from the opposite direction (**Figs. 8.4** and **8.5**).

- *Internal limiting membrane peeling*: This is a controversial area. Some believe that internal limiting membrane (ILM) removal removes a potential scaffold that can prevent recurrence of ERMs.

- Fluid–air exchange followed by gas injection may be done in cases with tractional retinal detachment.

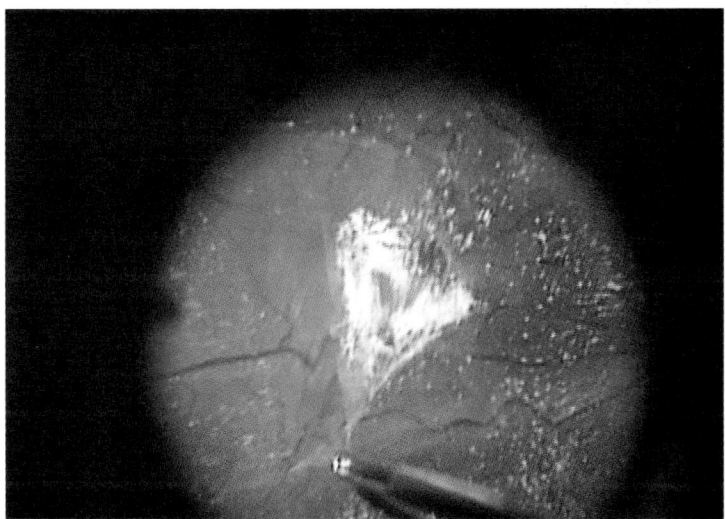

Fig. 8.2 Tangential traction applied on the membrane.

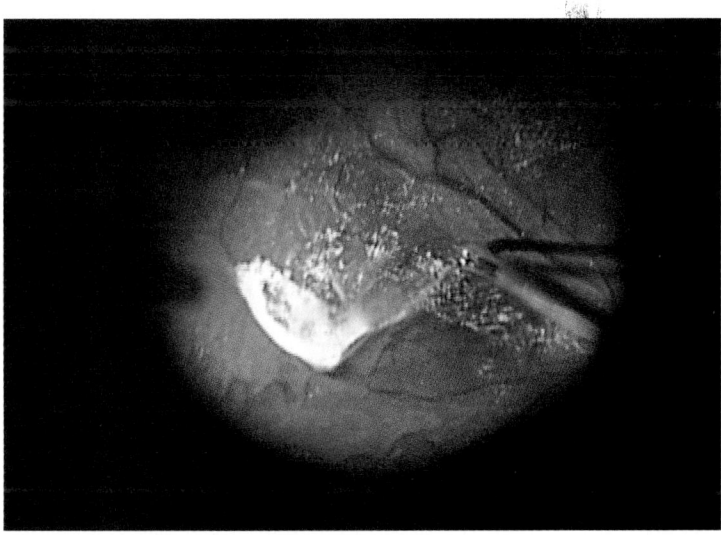

Fig. 8.3 Partially separated membrane.

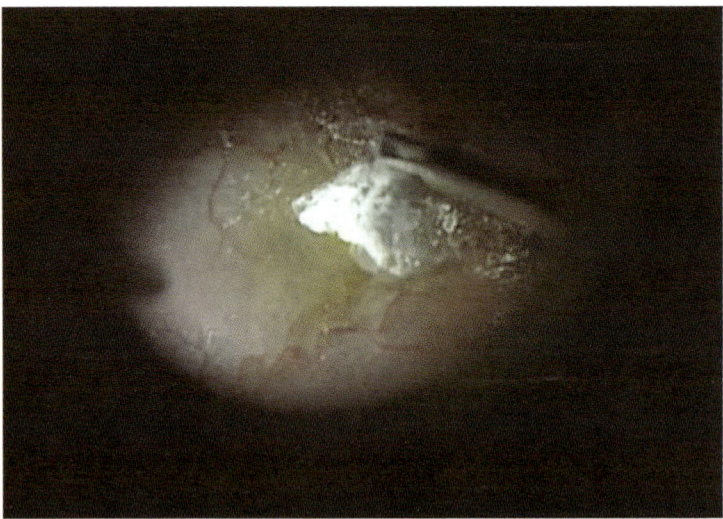

Fig. 8.4 Membrane grasped from different site due to strong adhesions.

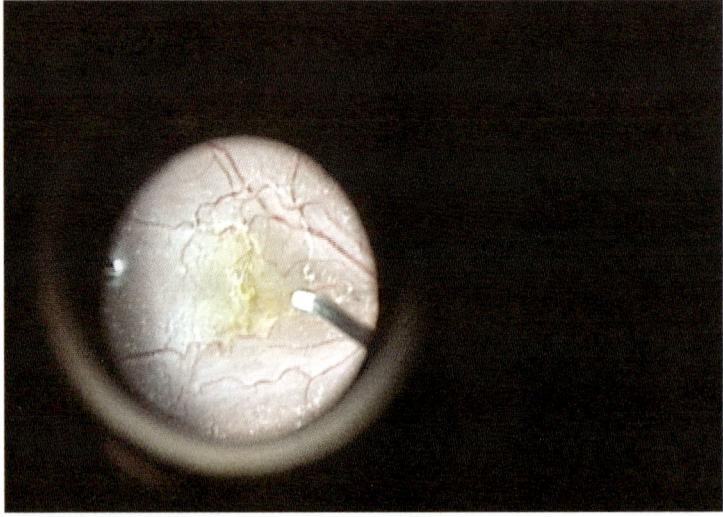

Fig. 8.5 Successfully removed membrane with distorted foveal architecture.

Macular Hole

While stage 3 and 4 holes have only surgical management, stage 2 holes may be followed up or operated upon, depending on presentation. Stage 1 holes are usually followed up. OCT is a useful tool for detection, documentation, prognostication, and locating associated findings such as epimacular membrane (EMM), CME, and VMT. Secondary causes include trauma, myopia, and diabetic macular edema (DME).

Visual results depend a lot on careful case selection. Prognostication is done on the basis of presenting visual acuity, stage of hole, cause of hole, associated ERM, and signs of chronicity. MH index and the Hole Form Factor being the most trusted indices. Informed consent should be taken and patient should be explained regarding the types of hole closure and hence the different prognoses. It is also important to explain to the patient the gradual improvement in vision which may take months.

Surgery for Macular Hole

- *PPV*: This is done for MH similarly to that for ERM. Similarly, triamcinolone-assisted PVD induction is done and peripheral vitrectomy is completed.

- *ILM peeling*: This is a must for stage 3 and stage 4 holes. The first challenge is visualization of the membrane itself. This is done with the help of dyes as in EMMs. While various dyes are available, indocyanine green has lost favor due to reports indicating that retinal pigment epithelium (RPE) and retinal phototoxicity are associated with it. Trypan blue stains the ILM only weakly, if at all, and requires contact time. BBG dye is perhaps the best available dye and does rapid and effective staining of the ILM. Dyes are also available in combination. ILM peeling as for ERMs can be done with the help of forceps. It is safer to begin from the temporal side of the fovea to avoid damage to the macular nerve fiber bundle. A small flap is raised (**Figs. 8.6** and **8.7**) and enlarged (**Figs. 8.8** and **8.9**) and first of all slid over the fovea (**Figs. 8.10** and **8.11**) as a whole to ensure that no tags are left near the edge of the hole itself. At this point, the edge of ILM is easily visible, and occurrence of any nerve fiber bleed essentially indicates the correct plane of peeling. Now another flap is raised or the first one held with forceps and peeling is performed in a circular manner to complete a "maculorhexis," just like capsulorhexis is done for cataract surgeries by repeated gripping of the membrane flap. Optimal size of the peel is debated but generally a size of one disc diameter is recommended.

- *Alternative techniques*: Nontraumatic instruments such as DDMS (**Figs. 8.12–8.16**) and soft-tip cannula may be used to lift the edge of the flap and later complete the membrane peel with forceps.

- *Fluid–air exchange (FAX)* is done in the routine way. At the end, a small-gauge, soft-tipped cannula may be used to dry out the edges of the hole to allow for better and quicker apposition of the hole edge (**Fig. 8.17**).

- *Gas injection* is usually done to keep the hole dry and allow closure. Only air may suffice in small stage 2 holes. Most holes close with a 3- to 7-day tamponade and the idea is to keep the hole out of contact with vitreous fluid. Prone position at least for 3 to 7 days is advisable especially if air or short-lasting gas is used to ensure dehydration of hole edges.

Inverted flap technique has been recently described for large MHs. In this technique, an inverted ILM flap is used for covering the MH bed followed by an extremely slow FAX.

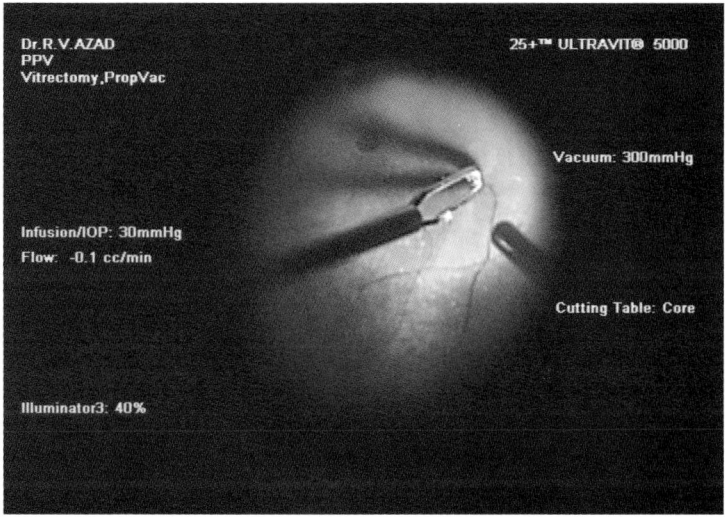

Fig. 8.6 Internal limiting membrane approached from temporal side with forceps.

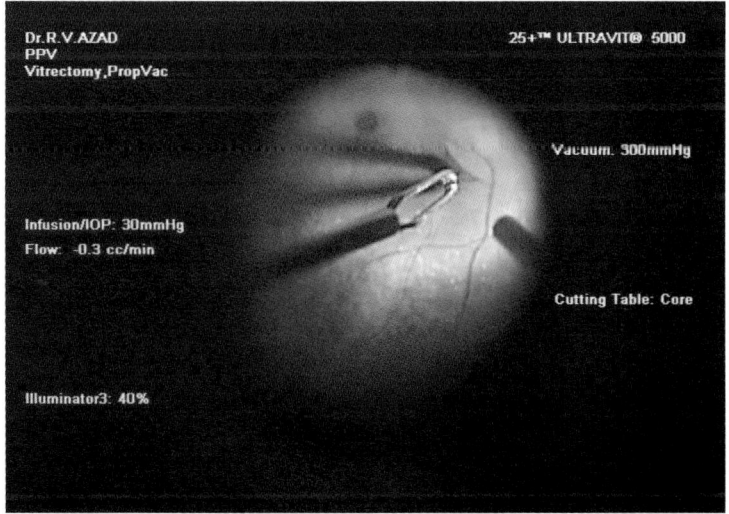

Fig. 8.7 Small internal limiting membrane flap raised.

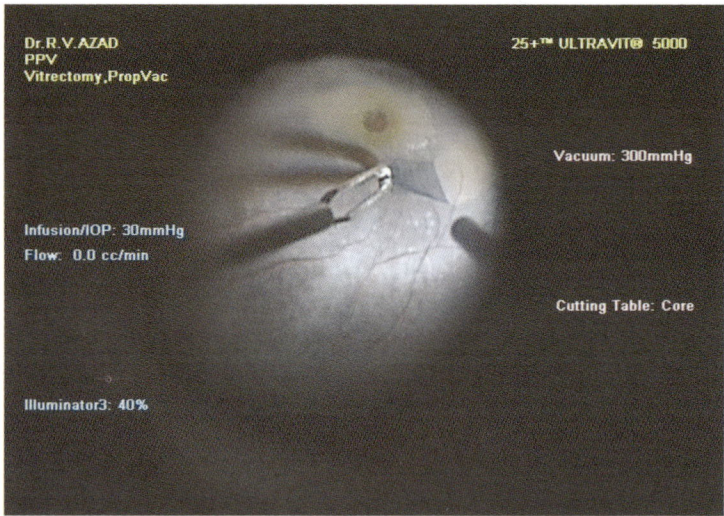

Fig. 8.8 Internal limiting membrane flap dragged tangentially.

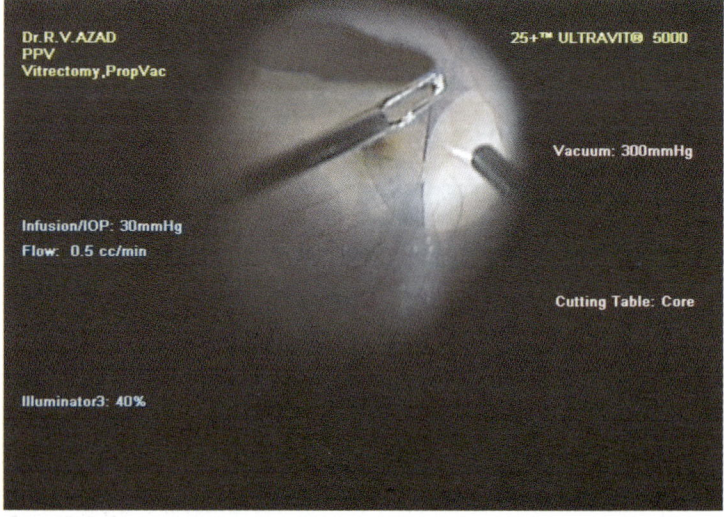

Fig. 8.9 Internal limiting membrane flap enlarged from the opposite side.

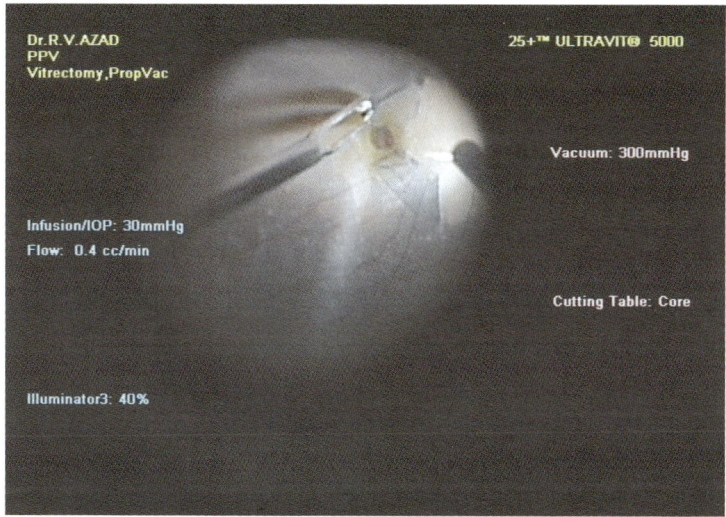

Fig. 8.10 Internal limiting membrane flap lifted tangentially across the macular hole.

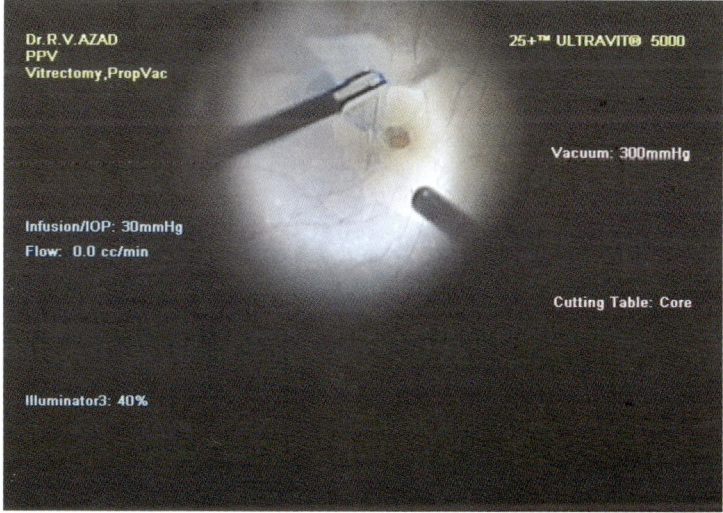

Fig. 8.11 No internal limiting membrane tags left at the edge of the hole.

109

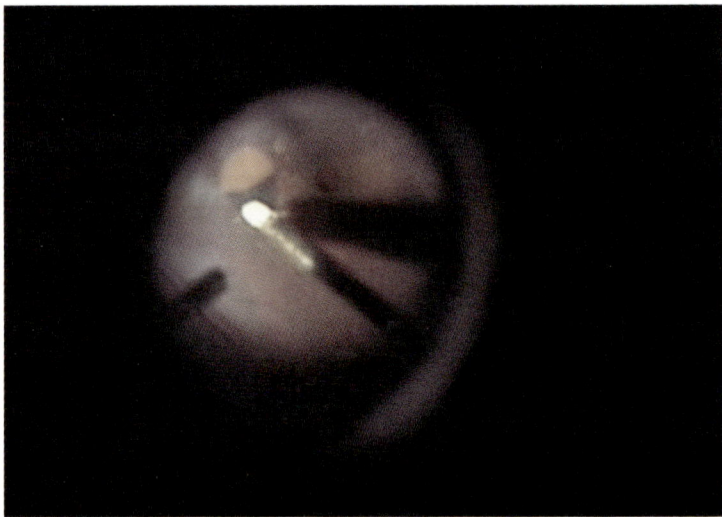

Fig. 8.12 Internal limiting membrane flap raised with diamond-dusted membrane scraper.

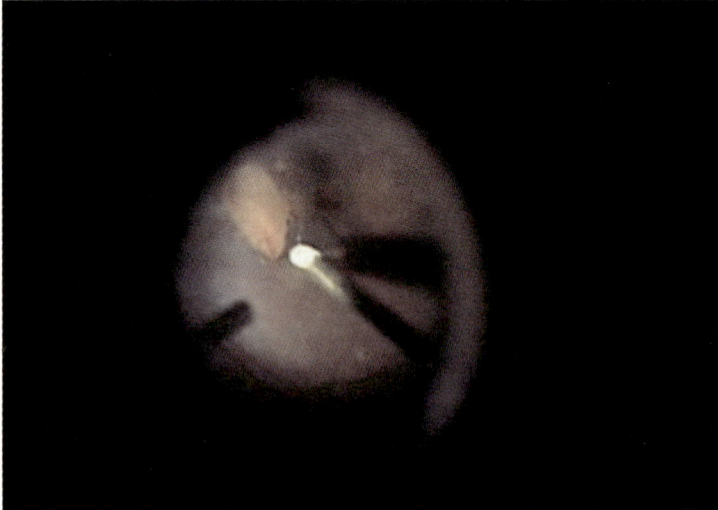

Fig. 8.13 Internal limiting membrane flap rolled tangentially with diamond-dusted membrane scraper.

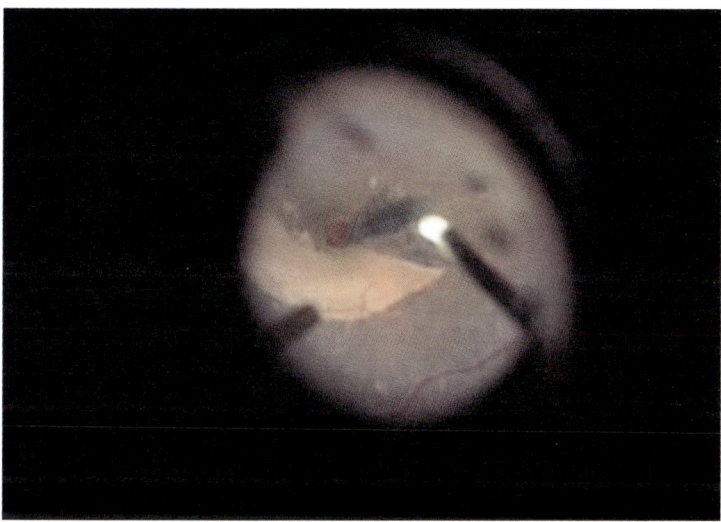

Fig. 8.14 Circumferential enlargement of the internal limiting membrane flap.

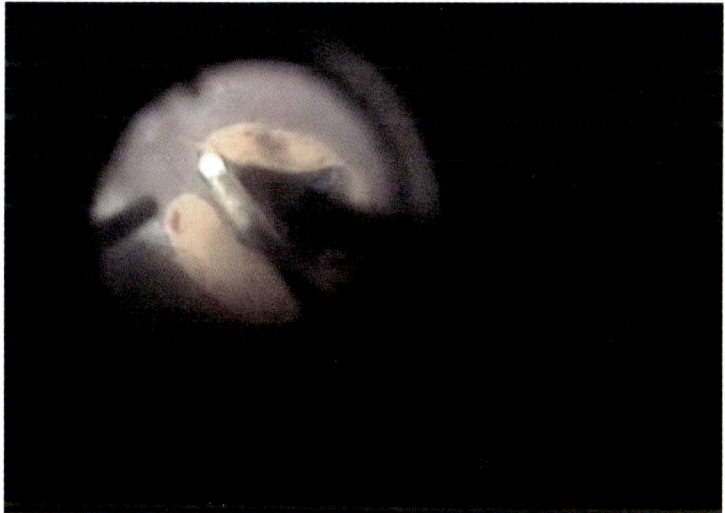

Fig. 8.15 Near-complete internal limiting membrane peel.

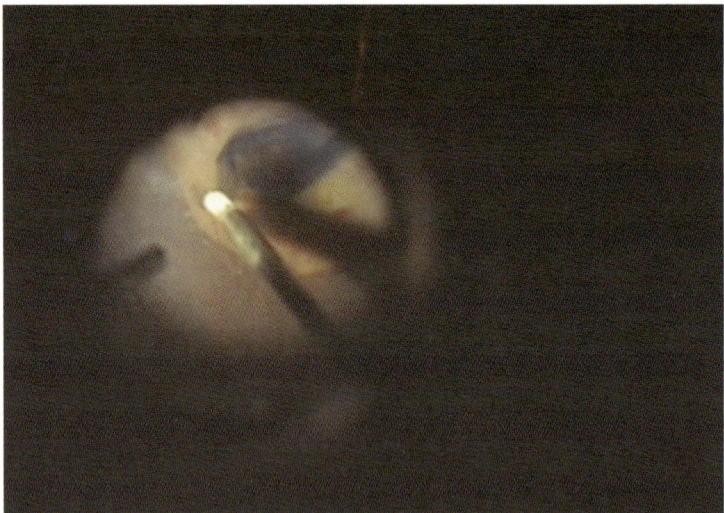

Fig. 8.16 Internal limiting being removed from the edge of the hole as the last step.

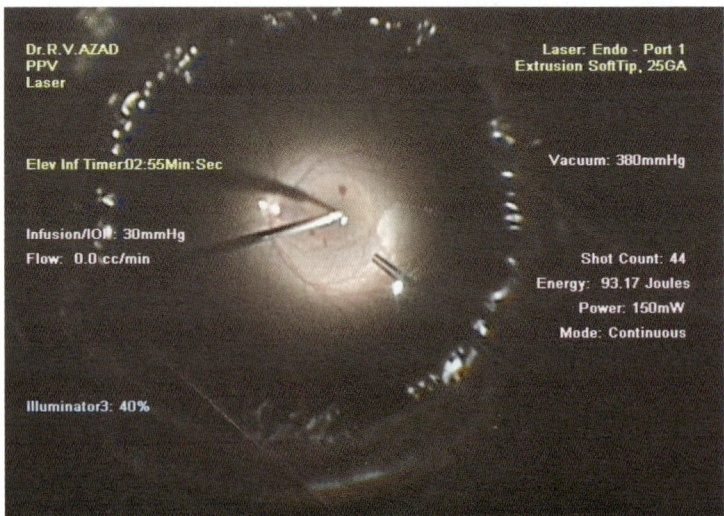

Fig. 8.17 Fluid–air exchange along with drying the edge of the hole.

Hole closure rates are as high as 90% especially in small holes. ILM peeling, gas tamponade, and postoperative positioning are essential in holes that have progressed beyond stage 2, while in stage 2 the choice is left to the surgeon.

Complications and Prognoses

Retinal detachment, endophthalmitis, cataract, glaucoma, ERMs, and other complications are common in any vitreous surgery and may compromise the benefits of a perfect surgery.

Specific to macular surgeries is the detection of visual field defects commonly inferotemporally, due to nasal PVD induction and FAX-related dehydration injury.

Recurrent ERMs may occur in around 20% of cases. These are more common in young patients.

Reopening of MH may occur in around 5 to 7% of the cases. Prognoses depends on presenting visual acuity, correct timing of surgery, and non-traumatic membrane peeling. OCT is invaluable in this regard. Visual recovery may take months to a year.

Vitreolysis is the latest available tool in macular surgeries but is under investigation. Other macular surgeries include surgery for VMT, CME-DME, macular/RPE translocation in age-related macular degeneration, and subretinal bleed management with intravitreal injections.

Surgical Tips

- ✓ Case selection and prognostication
- ✓ Triamcinolone acetonide–assisted hyaloid removal
- ✓ Dye selection for ERM/MH
- ✓ High-magnification and plano-concave lens for macular instrumentation
- ✓ Careful and nontraumatic membrane peeling
- ✓ Complete FAX in MH
- ✓ Gas tamponade and positioning with prior patient counseling

Nucleus Drop and Intraocular Lens Drop

*Brijesh Takkar and
Shorya Vardhan Azad*

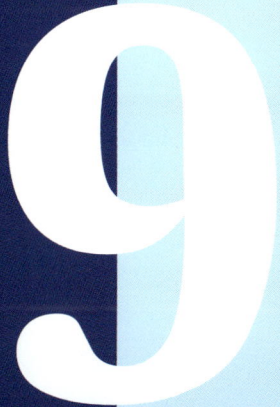

9 Nucleus Drop and Intraocular Lens Drop

Introduction

Management of nucleus drop and intraocular lens (IOL) drop starts with the anterior segment surgeon himself, in fact much before the surgery is started. Recognizing risk factors for such complications with patient counseling and arranging for vitrectomy backup allows for smooth management. However, if such a complication does occur, it is best if the anterior chamber is cleared of residual lens matter, good if anterior vitrectomy is performed, and, if anatomy permits, a posterior chamber IOL (PCIOL) is implanted and wound sutured good enough to provide a stable anterior chamber for posterior vitrectomy. With the modern-day vitrectomy setup, usually the dropped lens fragments are amenable to fragmentation and only if the nucleus is extremely hard, as seen in hyper mature senile cataract, levitation may be needed.

Preoperative Assessment

- *Work-up*: The surgeon should always be aware of the duration of the primary surgery, as it is an indicator of the strength since the primary surgical wound. The best visual potential of the eye should also be kept in mind, as it can alter surgical decisions and sometimes even the decision to operate. Corneal clarity is a must for surgery. While the presence of few Descemet's folds or only epithelial edema may not be a concern, surgery should be postponed if cornea is densely edematous. Next, anterior chamber should be evaluated for signs of inflammation, lens matter, or vitreous. Presence of hypopyon should be taken as an ominous sign and urgent management for endophthalmitis should be considered. Sometimes, vitreous or lens matter touch may lead to corneal edema, and first an anterior chamber cleanup may be required before embarking upon the vitreous surgery. Pupillary membranes may prevent complete dilatation. Capsular support for possible secondary IOL should be looked for. For nucleus drop, sclerosis of the other eyes' nucleus is a direct indicator of sclerosis of the dropped lens. Intraocular pressure (IOP) needs to be controlled as it is usually abnormal in such cases. Fundus visualization is difficult in dropped lens matter due to vitritis. One should carefully rule out retinal tears due to inadvertent vitreous traction, look for posterior vitreous detachment (PVD), and check whether lens matter/IOL is entangled in vitreous base, which requires careful manipulation during surgery. Again, all efforts should be made to rule out infective foci.

- *Indications for vitrectomy*: As per conventional training, nucleus matter of less than 25% and 2 mm or small cortical/epinuclear pieces may be left alone and the patient can be kept under follow-up. In most other situations, posterior segment intervention is needed. Similarly, regardless of the size, presence of glaucoma, uveitis, and cystoid macular edema (CME) warrant vitrectomy. The presence of endophthalmitis, vitreous hemorrhage, and retinal detachment (RD) also become obvious indications. Here, the role of the primary surgeon is important, as in presence of hazy media only he can estimate the amount of lens matter drop. In no case, however, fishing should be done as it is very dangerous and results in uncontrolled vitreous traction.

  Dropped IOLs should be removed especially if they are mobile and can potentiate retinal complications such as tears and RD. This holds true especially in those cases where PVD has not occurred. In some cases, the mobile IOL may obstruct vision by moving across the posterior pole, thereby necessitating its removal. Associated complications as mentioned earlier require surgery. Again, with the availability of safe and better instrumentation, perhaps all IOLs should be removed if a secondary IOL rehabilitation is planned, unless the patient or the patient's eye is not fit for surgery.

- *When to operate*: If setup and skilled surgeons are available, the surgery can be done immediately. In most cases, the cornea is clear immediately after surgery and hence posterior vitrectomy may be performed. If planned this way, the primary surgeon should remember not to hydrate the wound and fill the anterior chamber with a cohesive viscoelastic. Minor degrees of epithelial edema, however, can be managed with scraping or other similar techniques.

If the situation is converse, it is best to wait for at least 2 to 4 weeks for the acute inflammation to resolve and wound to gain good strength. One should remember to control the IOP and uveitis during this period. If uncontrolled and refractory glaucoma or uveitis persists, the surgeon may have to enter at the first available opportunity.

- *Placing the IOL:* If the IOL is not present already and best corrected visual acuity is good, the surgeon may decide to place the IOL in the same sitting. The choice of IOL, that is, scleral-fixated IOL, sulcus IOL, or anterior chamber (ACIOL), is decided by the usual rules as in any other patient. In the case of IOL drop, the surgeon should try to reposition the IOL or perform an IOL exchange depending upon individual expertise, the type of dropped IOL, and sulcus support. If needed, anterior segment surgeon's help may be taken. The best time to place the IOL during the surgery is when vitrectomy and fragmentation are complete and periphery has been examined. It should be done after temporarily securing the ports under fluid, and infusion pressure should be kept low to avoid iris prolapse as well as to maintain the eye volume.

Surgery for Nucleus Drop

Various surgeries have been described, including ultrasonic fragmentation, mechanical fragmentation, and levitation. Mostly, the lens fragments are amenable to ultrasonic fragmentation and rarely would a surgeon need to perform other techniques. Following steps are a guide to perform the surgery:

- *Gauge*: In the presence of hypotony or hazy media, which one may see after excessive anterior vitrectomy, long 20-gauge cannulas are the best. Otherwise, "hybrid" vitrectomy may be done where the surgeon starts with microinvasive vitrectomy surgery (MIVS) but enlarges the dominant port at the time of fragmentation as the probes for MIVS are not freely available. The infusion pressures should be adjusted accordingly.

- *PVD induction and complete peripheral vitrectomy* should be done after central vitrectomy to avoid retinal complications. Such complications can occur as in any other surgery but have a higher chance of occurring in fragmentation as a large bore instrument acting at high suction is introduced in the eye. Port-site dialysis can occur during its insertion. At the end of the surgery, one should therefore screen the port sites and peripheral retina with more care than usual and manage any adverse port-site events accordingly. If lens fragments are very soft or only cortical matter is present, one may get away with only vitrectomy and use the vitrector for removing the fragments with low cut rates and moderate to high suction.

- *PVD induction*: Inducing PVD is easy if the fragments are stuck in periphery and as most patients are elderly. Normal rules apply for the same. In such cases, it is better to do minimal core vitrectomy and then induce PVD first before going to periphery. Difficulty arises if the fragments are already on the posterior pole, as they constantly disturb the process by either obstructing the view or getting continuously entangled in the suction probe. In such a situation, one of the instruments should be aligned in such a way that it does not allow the nucleus to move and at the same time does not cause undue pressure on the posterior pole (**Fig. 9.1**).

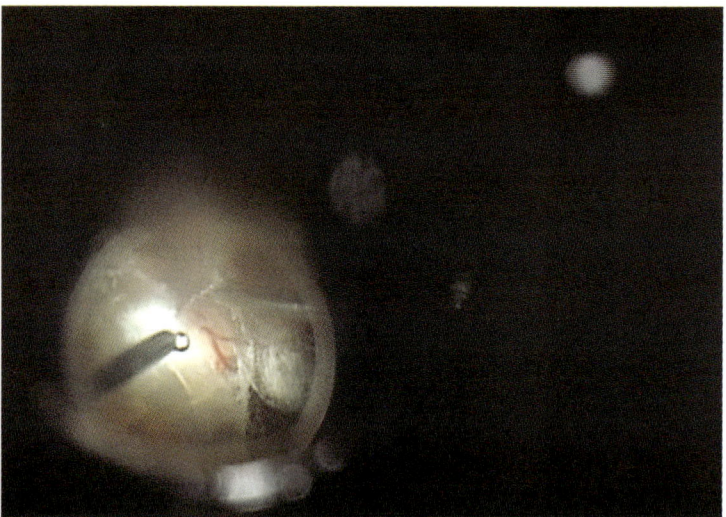

Fig. 9.1 Posterior vitreous detachment induction. The nucleus is controlled with the illuminator.

- *Perfluorocarbon liquid (PFCL)*: PFCLs are very helpful. They should be injected as soon as the PVD has been induced. The fragments thus float at the edge of the convex bubble, away from the visual area where suction can be applied easily (**Fig. 9.2**). Also in the event that the fragments fall from grip of the fragmentation probe, posterior pole would be partially protected. It should be aspirated at the end of the fragmentation.

- *Fragmentation*: Before introducing fragmatome, port sites should be checked for any residual vitreous which if found should be removed completely. One should remember the similarity of the process and probe with anterior phacoemulsification and apply the same principles during vitreous surgery. One should keep both the parameters, that is, phaco power and suction, to the minimum and then begin more controlled and complication-free surgery.

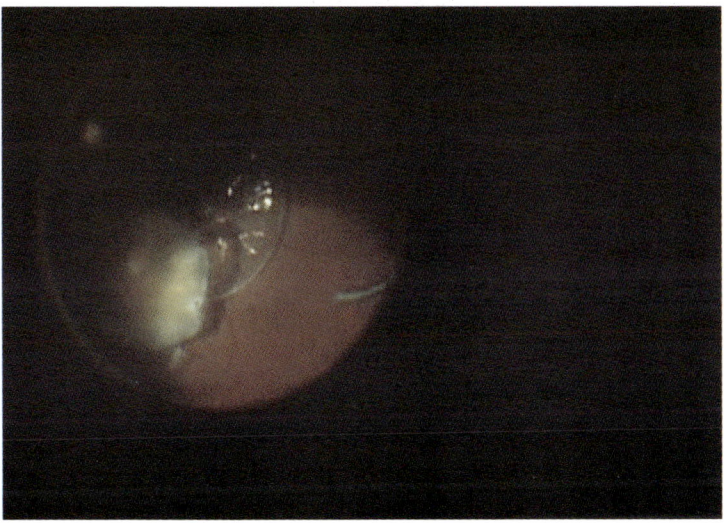

Fig. 9.2 Nucleus floating at the edge of the perfluorocarbon liquid bubble.

Suction usually needs to be increased. After applying adequate suction, the nucleus should be entangled in the probe and partially levitated to the midvitreous cavity (**Fig. 9.3**), and the fragmentation should be performed there so that retinal complications are minimal. The surgeon may use the second instrument or illuminator as a "chopping" instrument (**Fig. 9.4**). It is best not to remove the fragmentation probe till complete removal of the lens fragments has been done to avoid port-site events. Torsional phaco and pulse phaco have now been described in the posterior cavity as well. If one is dealing with large chunks of nucleus matter, one may observe these fragments to recurrently fall from the phaco probe on the posterior pole (**Fig. 9.5**). The surgeon should remain calm and remember to use minimal suction while lifting the fallen chunks and prolapsing them to the midvitreous cavity.

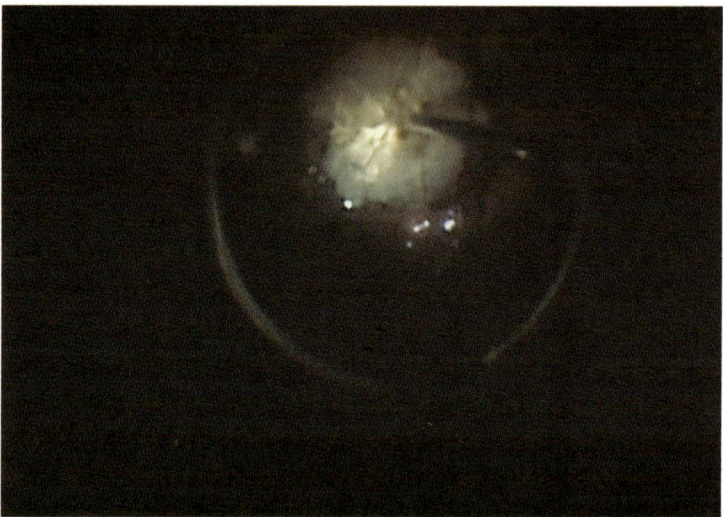

Fig. 9.3 Nucleus engaged with the cutter and prolapsed into the mid vitreous cavity.

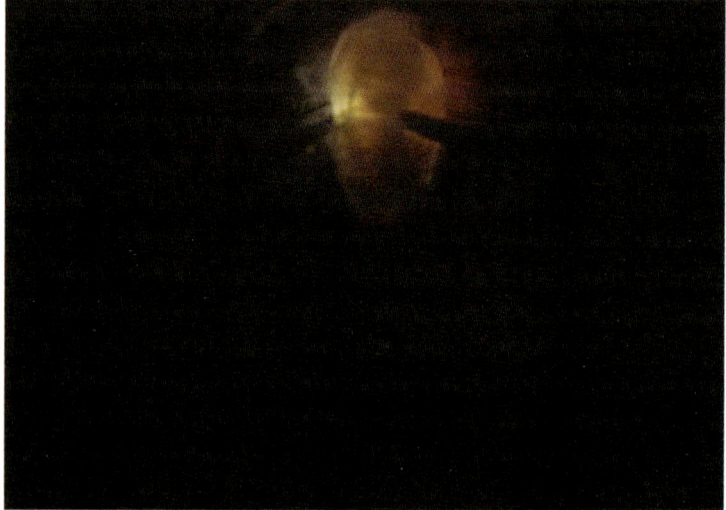

Fig. 9.4 The illuminator being used to divide the nucleus into smaller pieces.

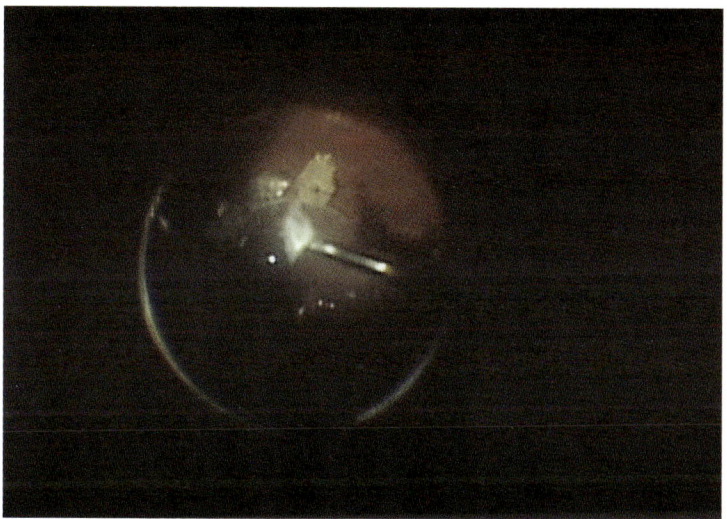

Fig. 9.5 Small nucleus fragments being emulsified.

- *If secondary IOL is planned*, this is the best time for the same. Ports should be closed. Infusion decreased to lower IOP that allow for the globe to remain formed and at the same time prevent the iris from prolapsing out of the wound. Then, ACIOL/sulcus IOL may be placed in a routine fashion. Wound should be closed tightly afterward and anterior chamber (AC) filled with viscocohesive or air so that IOL remains stable when fluid–air exchange (FAX) is performed.

- *Port closure*: A FAX may be performed as per surgeon's choice, and careful examination of the periphery should be done (**Fig. 9.6**). Any break found should be treated accordingly and endotamponade may be used as required. Routine precautions should be taken in aphakic patients. The heat energy of the fragmentation probe may desiccate and weaken the structure of the sclerotomy. One should hence be careful with the same and suture the port tightly.

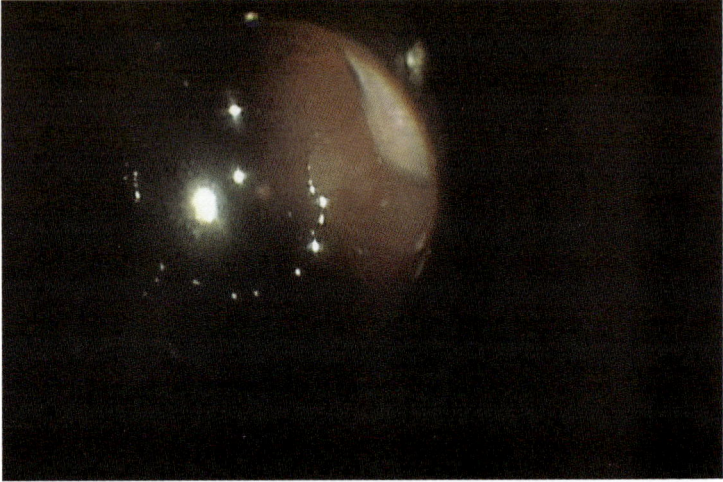

Fig. 9.6 Retinal periphery being indented and examined for retinal breaks.

Surgery for Intraocular Lens Drop

Largely, the surgery remains the same as described earlier till PVD induction, for the following differences:

- *Grasping the IOL*: Vitreous surrounding the IOL should be completely dissected and the IOL disengaged from it (**Fig. 9.7**). PFCL may be injected to levitate the IOL edge away from retina for easier grasping (**Fig. 9.8**). While grasping the IOL, the best instrument to use is the end-gripping forceps. If one is planning to explant the IOL, the nursing staff should be ready with the instruments required for making the limbus incision and extraction of the IOL. In this situation, it is best to hold at the haptic-optic junction (**Fig. 9.9**) and prolapse the IOL anteriorly. Care should be taken not to entangle the distal haptic in any ocular structure, and capsular remnants should be protected for future implantation of IOLs. The assistant may be asked

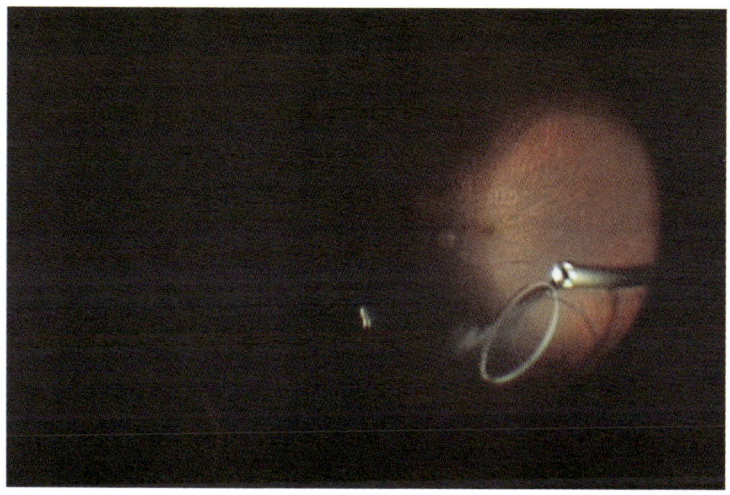

Fig. 9.7 Dislocated intraocular lens being freed from vitreous adhesions.

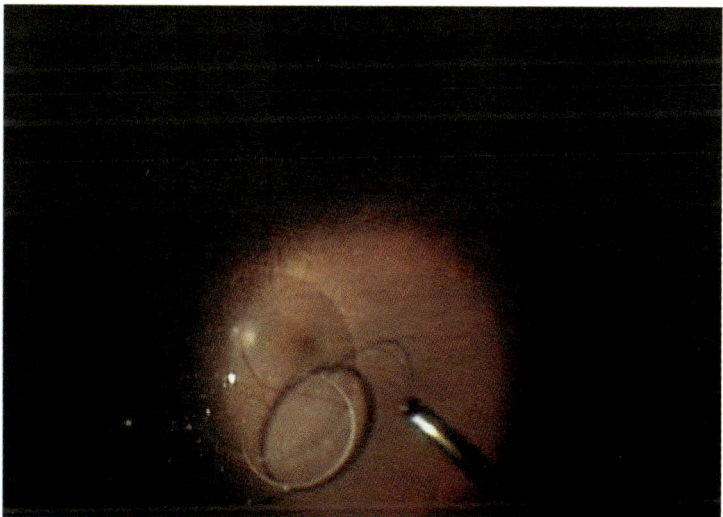

Fig. 9.8 Intraocular lens resting on the convexity of the perfluorocarbon liquid bubble.

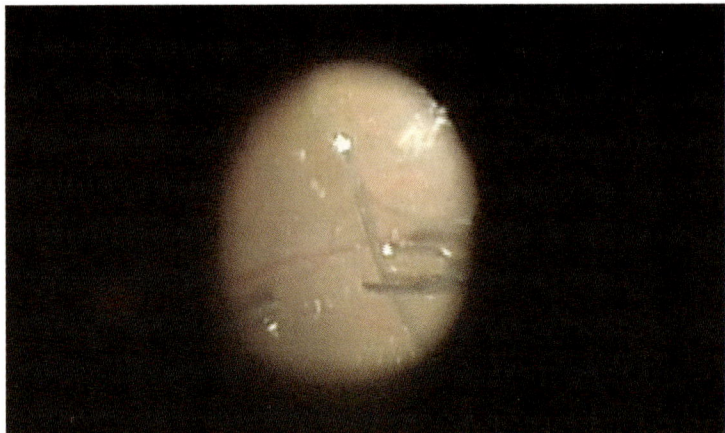

Fig. 9.9 Intraocular lens being gripped at the optic-haptic junction with forceps.

here to make an adequate-sized limbus incision superiorly (**Fig. 9.10**) (if comfortable, the surgeon may do the same with nondominant hand) and a second instrument should be used to gently prolapse the IOL from the limbus, keeping the wound safe (**Fig. 9.11**). Then the wound should be carefully sutured and surgery completed.

- *Repositioning*: If IOL repositioning is planned, the surgeon should preplan where to grip the IOL from. The best is to prolapse the IOL anteriorly in the previous manner and then use second forceps or a Sinskey hook and implant the distal haptic in the sulcus so that it faces leftward. Then the second haptic is aligned by reverse dialing and later the optic is positioned. One may use two Sinskey hooks for final adjustment of the IOL.

After finishing, the postoperative care is usual and steroids should be used judiciously to manage and prevent CME seen commonly after surgery. Visual outcomes are good in uncomplicated surgeries.

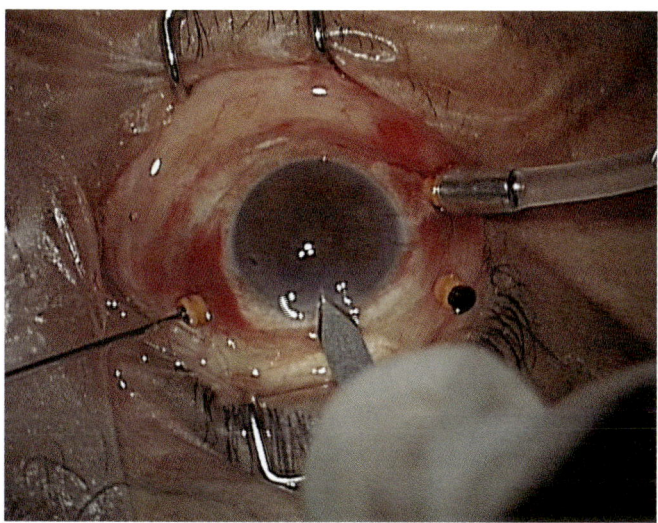

Fig. 9.10 Corneal incision being made at the limbus for removal of the intraocular lens.

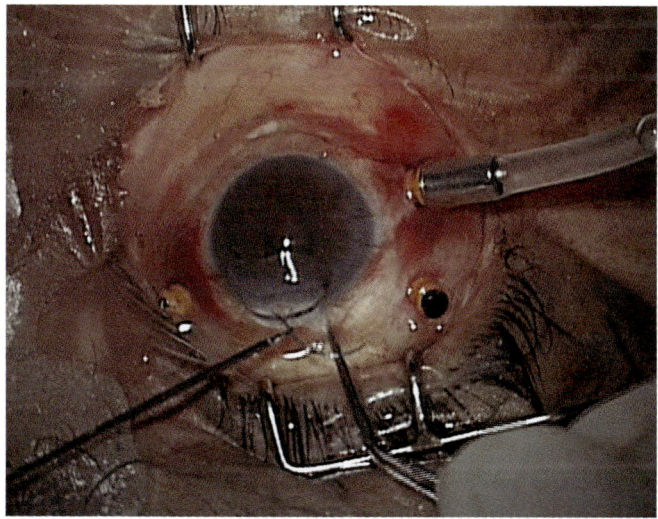

Fig. 9.11 Intraocular lens being delivered at the limbus.

Complications and Prognoses

Uneventful surgery usually has good visual prognoses, especially if the cataract surgery had not caused corneal problems. Important complications include macular edema, retinal tears, retinal detachment, and glaucoma. A meticulous approach, however, prevents as well as allows for better management of such complications.

Surgical Tips

- ✓ Observation and no surgery in selected few cases
- ✓ Managing uveitis and glaucoma
- ✓ PVD induction and complete posterior vitrectomy
- ✓ Careful handling of the fragmentation probe
- ✓ Peripheral retinal examination

Retained Intraocular Foreign Body

Brijesh Takkar and Shorya Vardhan Azad

10

10 Retained Intraocular Foreign Body

Introduction

Surgical removal of intraocular foreign body (IOFB) is perhaps the most unpredictable surgery, especially in the presence of media haze, requiring intense preoperative work-up and patient counseling. Typically, the patients are males, aged 20 to 40 years. Traditionally, glass/inert metal particles and clean stone particles, and even a subset of metallic foreign bodies, were managed conservatively. However, with the advent of modern-day vitrectomy systems, conservative management is largely avoided due to the lifelong risk of metallosis and endophthalmitis.

Preoperative Assessment

Work-up: After performing a comprehensive routine work-up and determining the type of foreign body, the surgeon should lay special emphasis first on the entry wound and decide if resuturing of surgical wound is required. Next, all efforts should be made to rule out endophthalmitis, as this becomes a surgical emergency of the utmost nature. Precise localization of the foreign body should be done along with estimation of its size by comparing it with optic disc. Encapsulation should be looked for as it requires special surgical maneuvers. If the foreign body is not visible due to cataract, hemorrhage, or exudates, radio imaging should be done. While X-ray should be ordered in all the cases for medicolegal documentation, ultrasound goes a long way in localizing the foreign body in the layers of the eye and noncontrast computed tomography (NCCT) should be done when sonography is nonconclusive. If in doubt as to the location of the foreign body in the external coats or outside the eye, NCCT should be ordered. Ultrasonography is also essential in ruling out retinal detachments (RDs) and exudation.

Patient counseling: Pars plana vitrectomy (PPV) for IOFB has endless number of complications and hence counseling is very important. Foreign bodies lying at the posterior pole or near the optic nerve head (ONH) carry very grave prognoses. Similarly, IOFB with RD, endophthalmitis, and siderosis has very poor prognoses. The patient should always be explained the risk of posterior pole impact site, the possibility of the foreign body being left in situ, especially if larger part is external. Consent for pars plana lensectomy (PPL) must be taken in case only limbal removal is possible.

Surgery

IOFBs should be removed as soon as possible. Earlier, anterior subchoroidal/subretinal foreign bodies of the posterior segment were removed via the external route. Also, small metallic foreign bodies with clear media were removed with extraocular (EO) magnets kept at the port without vitrectomy. Studies from our center have suggested that vitrectomy has better results with encirclage than without.

- Wound should be secured if open or weakly apposed. Encirclage, if planned, should be placed in the routine fashion.

- A standard three-port pars plana vitrectomy (PPV) is done. Conventionally, 20-gauge surgeries have been preferred, but these days microinvasive vitrectomy surgery (MIVS) is being performed with equally good results. It should be remembered that both foreign body forceps and intraocular (IO) magnets require 19-gauge ports; hence, the port sites need to be extended, which is easily done in MIVS.

- Central vitrectomy should be done, and if the foreign body/capsule is impacted in the retina or there are other retinal breaks, the surgeon may choose to laser these areas before inducing the posterior vitreous detachment (PVD). Triamcinolone-assisted PVD induction is performed and small foreign bodies located at the vitreoretinal interface are often seen to move along with the posterior hyaloid (**Figs. 10.1** and **10.2**).

- Perfluorocarbon liquid (PFCL) should be injected over the macula as soon as PVD is induced to avoid subretinal bleed at the macula and decrease the traumatic impact of a foreign body falling on the macula at the time of removal.

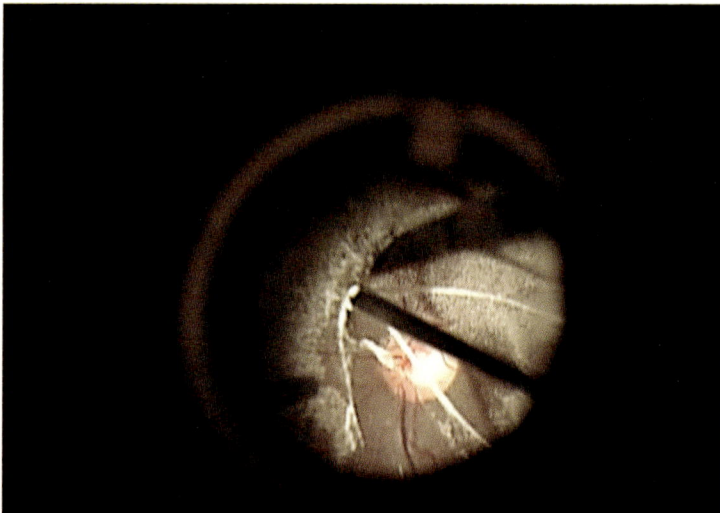

Fig. 10.1 Triamcinolone-stained posterior hyaloid.

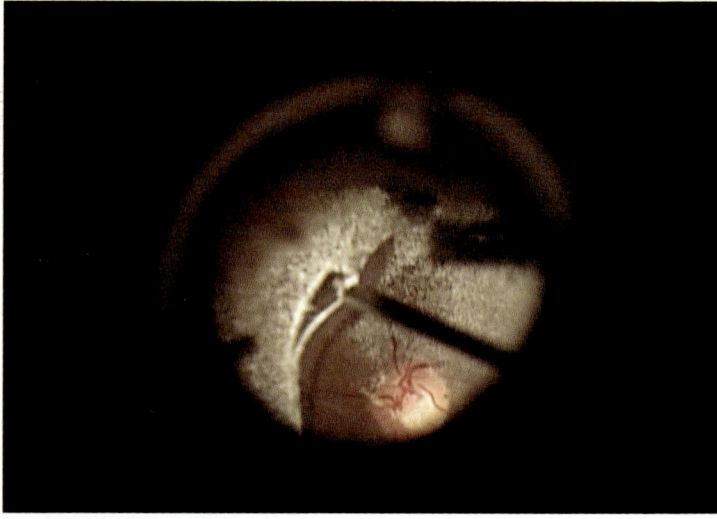

Fig. 10.2 Posterior vitreous detachment being induced from the nasal side.

- All vitreous surrounding the foreign body should be removed before embarking on IOFB removal (**Figs. 10.3** and **10.4**). Encapsulated foreign body can be removed together with the capsule (**Fig. 10.5**). However, in presence of fibrotic adhesions seen with longstanding foreign bodies, the capsule requires to be incised with the help of either the vitrectomy cutter or MVR blade knives to create an opening large enough to allow prolapse of the foreign body. Port-site vitrectomy should also be done meticulously.

- *Localizing the IOFB*: While most often the IOFBs can be easily seen, sometimes in hazy media such as in endophthalmitis or anterior foreign bodies, this may be very difficult. At this time, radio imaging should be referred to and the eye should be carefully scanned for the IOFB. Scleral indentation should be done and even elective PPL in clear

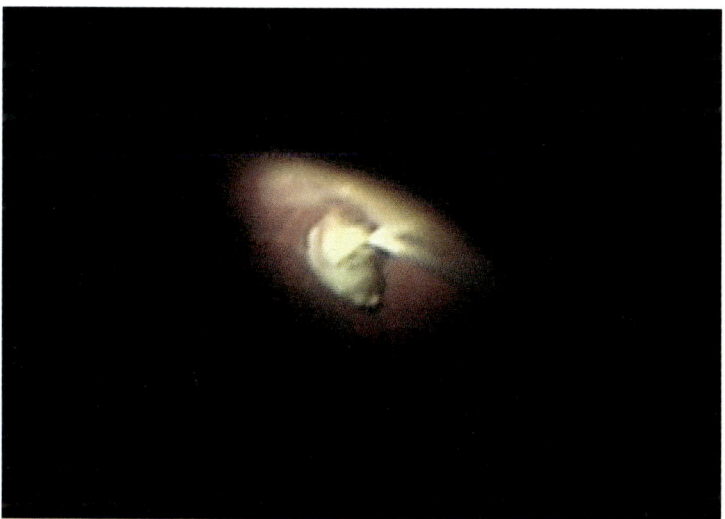

Fig. 10.3 Foreign body being freed from capsulo-vitreal adhesions.

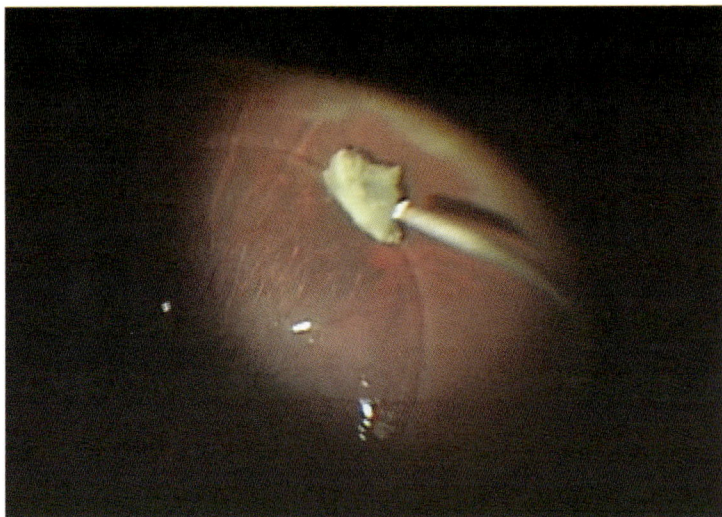

Fig. 10.4 Foreign body at the edge of the perfluorocarbon liquid bubble.

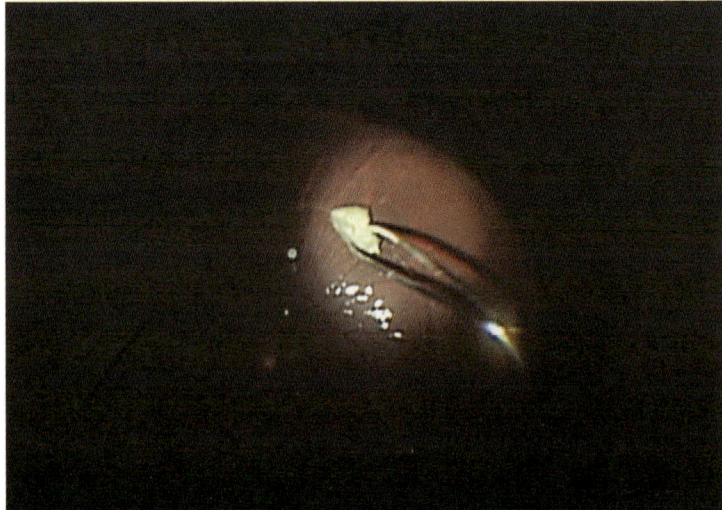

Fig. 10.5 Foreign body grasped with forceps.

lens should be considered in the event of anterior foreign bodies lodged in the pars plana. It is very important to have patience and not to panic.

- *Extraction of the IOFB*: This is a very crucial step associated with numerous complications. Metallic foreign bodies can be removed with the help of IO and EO magnets. After enlarging the scleral wound with MVR knife sufficient for a 19-gauge instrument, the intraocular magnet is introduced in the eye and the foreign body is directly grasped with the magnetic pull. Then the magnet is withdrawn slowly toward the scleral site under direct vision where the assistant places the stronger EO magnet at the margin of the sclerotomy. Thin and small foreign bodies can be easily removed; however, it is advisable to enlarge the sclerotomy site further and even introduce an additional instrument in the sclerotomy to keep its mouth wide open to allow safe removal of the IOFB. In the event of the foreign body getting stuck at the port, the surgeon should not panic as most often the metallic foreign body would still be entangled in the ciliary body due to the strong pull of the extraocular magnet and can be safely extracted by gentle instrumentation and maneuvering the magnet itself. Similar steps can be followed if limbus is the chosen site for removal. If the IOFB slips back into the vitreous cavity during the procedure, the surgeon may repeat the steps carefully or opt for foreign body forceps.

Nonmagnetic foreign bodies require removal with forceps. Various forceps are available now. Most commonly, diamond-coated straight forceps are used. The surgeon should first enlarge the wound site suitable for the forceps. These forceps are introduced and opened up only when sufficiently near the foreign body. Attempt should be made to grasp the foreign body in a way that allows for easiest removal. This can be done with the help of illuminator by aligning the IOFB such that the thinnest part of the IOFB is removed through the sclerotomy site, hence being minimally destructive. Practically, it should be remembered that the forceps often get magnetized if kept close to the magnets, which makes maneuverability difficult, and also that the sleeve can get stuck, so it is best to check for smoothness of the instrument before introducing inside the eye. Port-site vitreous frequently gets entangled in this sleeve of the forceps, so it is best if recurrent opening and closing is avoided. Removal of the IOFB can be performed safely as described earlier (apart from the use of magnets). If successful alignment cannot be performed or the IOFB gets stuck recurrently at the port site, "handshake" technique may be applied where another forceps is introduced from the opposite port to grasp the IOFB in anterior vitreous cavity for removal.

During extraction, the surgeon should remember that since the sclerotomy has been enlarged, the globe tends to collapse due to hypotony. The infusion pressure hence should be increased and the sclerotomy should be sutured partially as soon as the foreign body has been removed. The IOFB should then be safely preserved and handed over to the patient for medicolegal purposes/patient satisfaction (**Figs. 10.5–10.9**).

- After extracting the IOFB, careful inspection of the port sites should be done to look for possible port-site events or dialysis (**Fig. 10.10**) and they should be managed accordingly. All full-thickness retinal breaks should be treated with laser retinopexy.

- The surgeon may opt to complete the fluid-air exchange (FAX) and may perform gas or oil injection as per requirement.

- The ports and peritomy are then closed and routine postoperative care is prescribed.

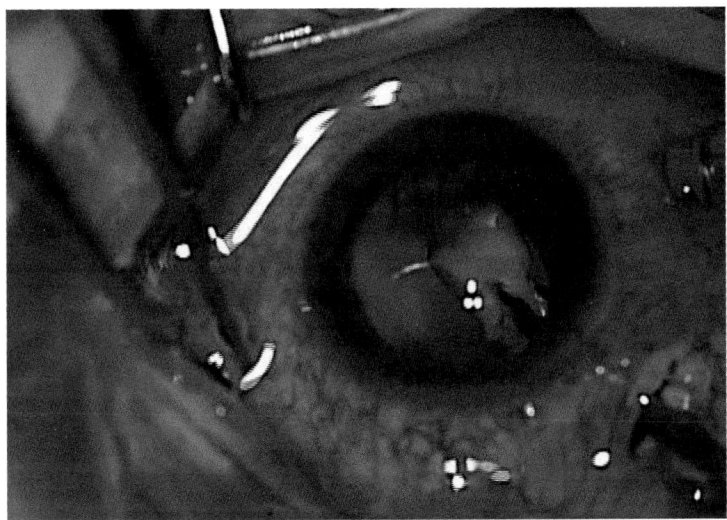

Fig. 10.6 Foreign body prolapsed into the anterior vitreous cavity.

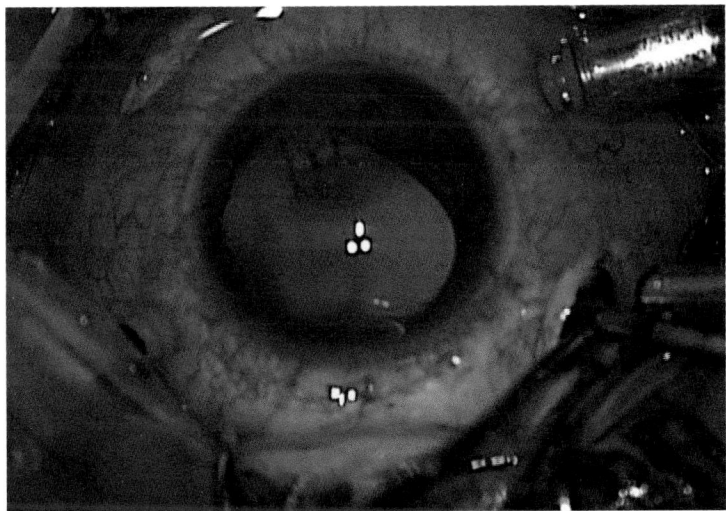

Fig. 10.7 Foreign body being delivered through an enlarged sclerotomy bimanually. Note the tip of the extraocular magnet at the posterior lip of sclerotomy.

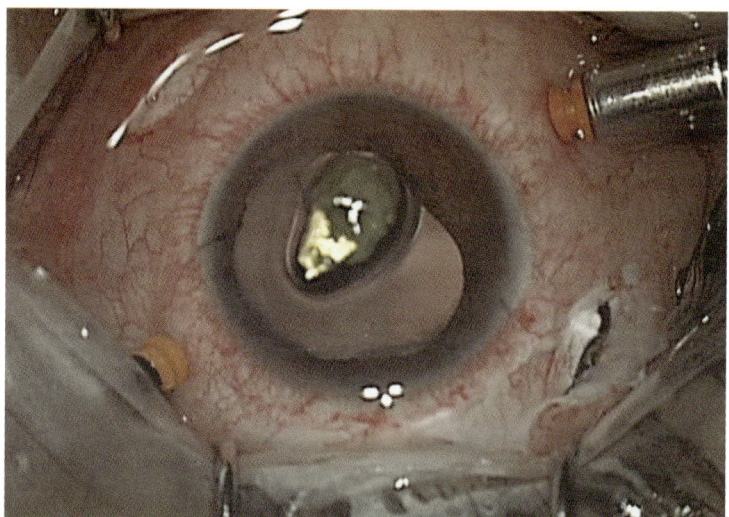

Fig. 10.8 Externalized foreign body.

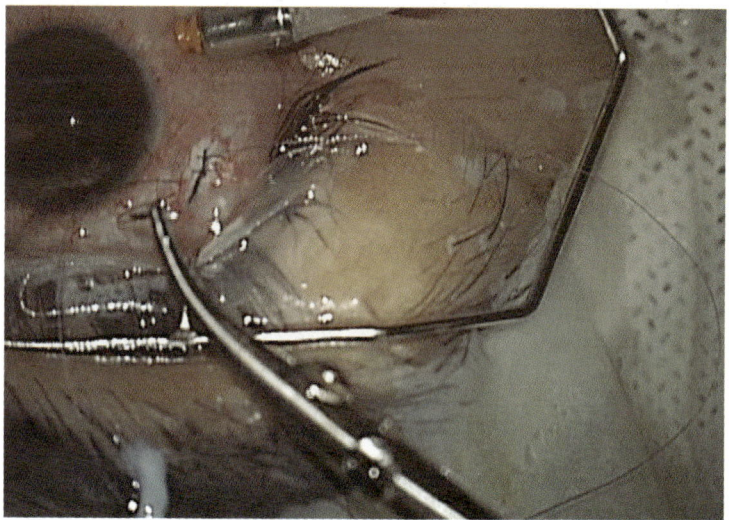

Fig. 10.9 Partial suture-assisted closure of the sclerotomy site.

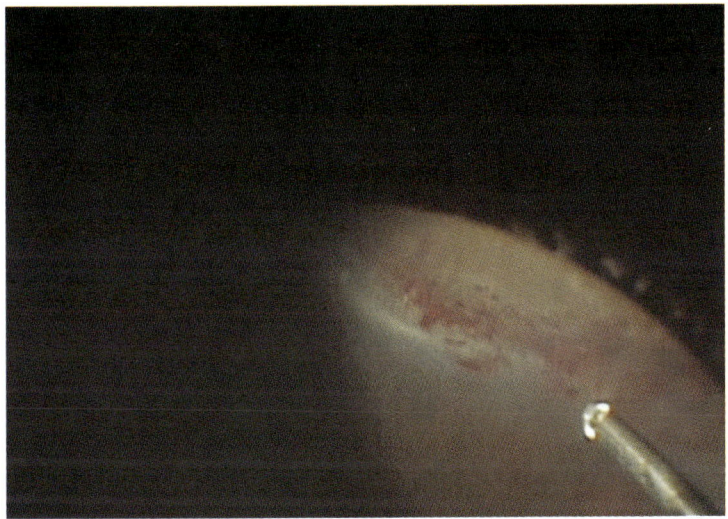

Fig. 10.10 Peripheral and port-site indentation examination for retinal breaks.

Complications and Prognoses

Leaving aside all the general complications of PPV, intraoperatively the IOFB may fall from grasp of the forceps and injure the posterior pole, leading to irreversible complications. Hypotony-related and port-site complications are much more frequent than in other surgeries. Similarly, intraoperative RDs are known to occur and lens touch can occur during extraction of a large IOFB. Even successful and uneventful removal of IOFBs can be complicated in the postoperative period by RDs, metallosis, endophthalmitis, PVR changes, cataract, and glaucoma, to name a few. Hence, patient should be cautioned for a guarded visual prognosis in every case of IOFB.

Surgical Tips

- ✓ Careful and complete work-up with precise localization
- ✓ Management of the wound site and optimum timing of the surgery
- ✓ Port site and complete vitrectomy followed by dissection of the IOFB from traction/capsule
- ✓ Safe and slow extraction followed by inspection of the port sites
- ✓ Patient counseling as complications are expected

Endophthalmitis

Shorya Vardhan Azad and
Brijesh Takkar

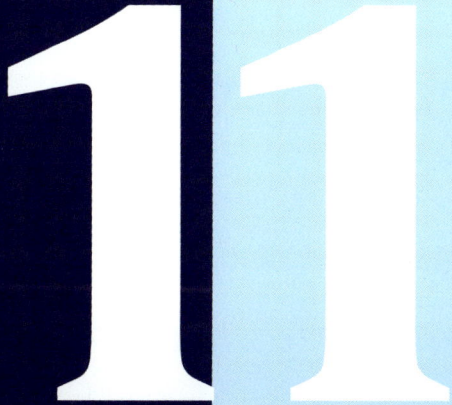

11

11 Endophthalmitis

Introduction

Endophthalmitis is an inflammation of the inner coats of the eye. The most important cause is postoperative infection, followed by others such as post-traumatic and endogenous infection. Apart from Endophthalmitis Vitrectomy Study (EVS), which guides management for post–cataract surgery acute bacterial infection, there is no other high-level evidence trial for management for delayed/traumatic/endogenous/other postoperative endophthalmitis. One should rule out panophthalmitis before deciding for surgery.

Preoperative Assessment

Work-up: Recording the visual acuity, intraocular pressure (IOP), neovascularization of iris, and vitreous opacification is important, as these indicate chronicity and severity of infection. Managing the anterior segment is a big bugbear in itself. In postoperative cases, one should also look for the status of the primary surgical wound, as it may need suturing before beginning the surgery. Also in cases where scleral tunnels have been employed, one may see tunnel infection which present predominantly with anterior segment signs. Corneal status is also of importance in providing media for surgery. While corneal abscess or frank keratitis may require a corneal surgery as well, cornea is usually found decompensated with Descemet's folds, or stromal edema, or keratic precipitates, regardless of the IOP status, due to the ongoing intense inflammation. One may also see pupillary membranes which often require removal. Use of intravitreal antibiotics and steroids may decrease the inflammation and make the surgery easier.

Sonography is of immense importance as around 15% of the cases may have retinal detachment (RD). These may be shallow/bullous and rhegmatogenous/exudative. Their presence is an indication for surgery, and further declines the visual prognoses. One may localize choroidal detachments in the inflamed and hypotonous eye, which guides the placement of infusion cannula.

Indication for surgery: The difference in management in different settings is not only due to the inciting event but also due to the difference in microbial etiology seen in these cases. Organisms causing acute postoperative bacterial endophthalmitis are differently virulent and sensitive to antibiotics. For example, while gram-positive micrococci such as *Staphylococcus* species cause postcataract acute infections, in delayed cases a large proportion is shared by organisms such as *Propionibacterium acnes* and fungi-like *Candida/Aspergillus*. Similarly, post–filtration surgery streptococci are causative, while in posttraumatic infections *Bacillus* and gram-negative microbes play an important role. Scenario in endogenous endophthalmitis depends on source of infection but usually gram-negative microbes and fungi from integumentary, gastrointestinal, and urinary tracts are common. This partly explains the differences.

As per the EVS, in acute bacterial post–cataract surgery endophthalmitis with presenting visual acuity below hand movement close to face (accurate projection of rays), vitrectomy has better long-term visual prognoses in comparison to medical management. In *P. acnes* endophthalmitis, vitrectomy along with membranectomy , ± In the bag vancomycin wash +/- intraocular lens (IOL)-bag explant, is usually required. Similarly, delayed/ fungal and posttraumatic endophthalmitis cases also usually require early surgical intervention. Post–filtration surgery, blebitis patients can be managed medically, but in endophthalmitis, vitrectomy is indicated. In endogenous cases, although systemic antibiotics have a huge role, vitrectomy gives the advantage of obtaining a large sample size for microbial cultures. In fact, vitrectomy is said to have three times better anatomical and functional outcomes as against conservative management in endogenous cases.

Counseling and consult: Visual prognosis remains extremely guarded in this setting of compartmentalized infection of the globe. The risk of recurrence of infections in fungal and *P. acnes* cases is alarming. Indolent fungal infections can lead to painful phthisis despite a good surgery. Risk of panophthalmitis and intracranial infections should also be explained. Consent should also be taken for requirement of repeat surgery in the event of RD, recurrent infection, oil removal, cataract, etc.

Surgery

Endophthalmitis is one of the most difficult cases for the ophthalmic surgeon. Patience is the key.

- *Encirclage*: A scleral band in infected cases has the disadvantage of possible spread of the infection and excessive bleeding of the inflamed tissue. However, one may opt for it in cases such as RD with intraocular foreign body and endophthalmitis where adequate vitrectomy is impossible without complications.

- *Gauge*: In the presence of choroidal detachment (CD) and unknown retinal status, 20-gauge vitrectomy is perhaps the safest and most preferred, although microinvasive vitrectomy surgery (MIVS) may be safely used in pseudophakic/aphakic patients.

- *Placing the infusion cannula*: 6-mm cannulas should be used when pars plana lensectomy is planned or in pseudophakia to avoid the severe risk of subretinal/suprachoroidal cannulas. The irrigation should not be switched on till one is absolutely sure of the status of the cannula (**Fig. 11.1**). One may either place anterior chamber (AC) maintainers (**Fig. 11.2**) or infusion through the pars plana route especially if the anterior vitreous allows its monitoring in the pupillary plain. The AC may be cleared with viscoelastics/cutter/blunt dissection (**Figs. 11.3–11.7**). Exudates behind the IOL should be removed (**Fig. 11.8**), and sometimes IOL explants may be necessary. The main infusion should be switched on only when the media allows and the surgeon is sure of the correct position of cannula.

- *IOL explant*: This may be required in *P. acnes* endophthalmitis and unstable IOLs.

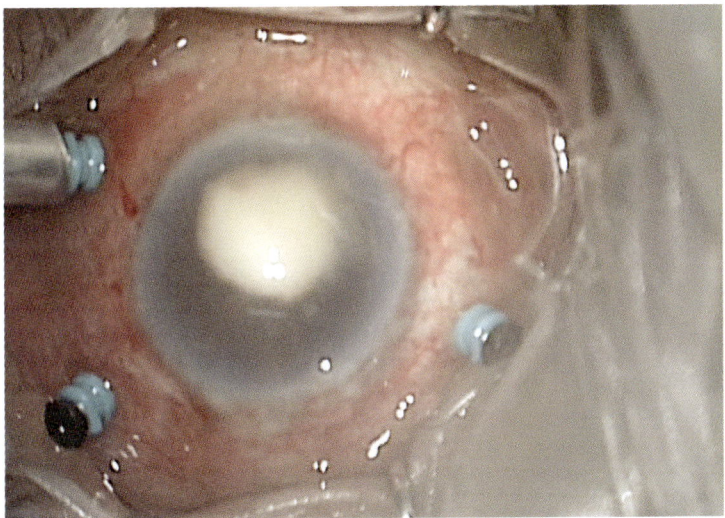

Fig. 11.1 Hazy cornea with exudates in anterior chamber not allowing visualization of the inserted infusion cannula.

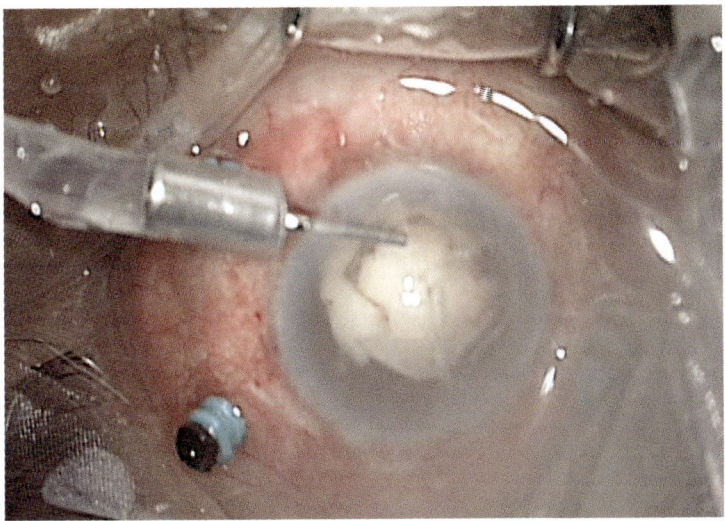

Fig. 11.2 The infusion cannula being used as an anterior chamber maintainer.

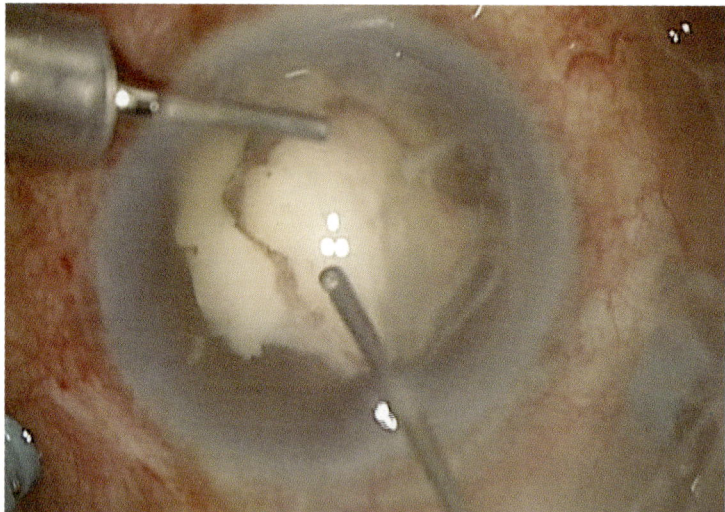

Fig. 11.3 Cutter inserted into anterior chamber through limbus-based incision after failed viscodissection.

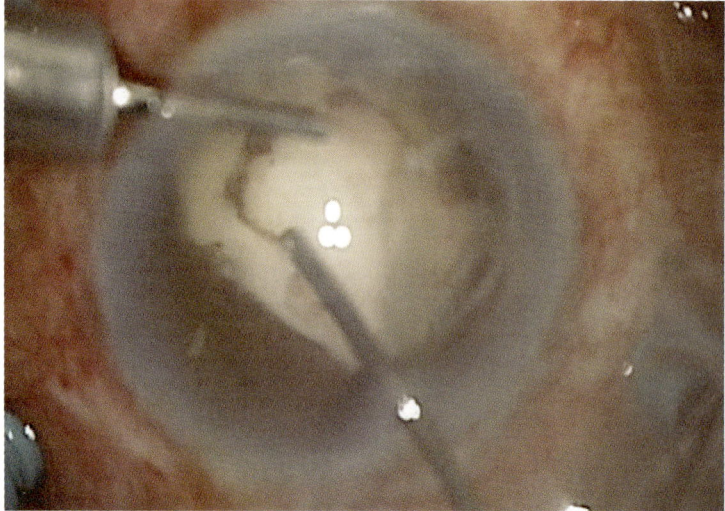

Fig. 11.4 Cutter being used to free the exudates from the iris.

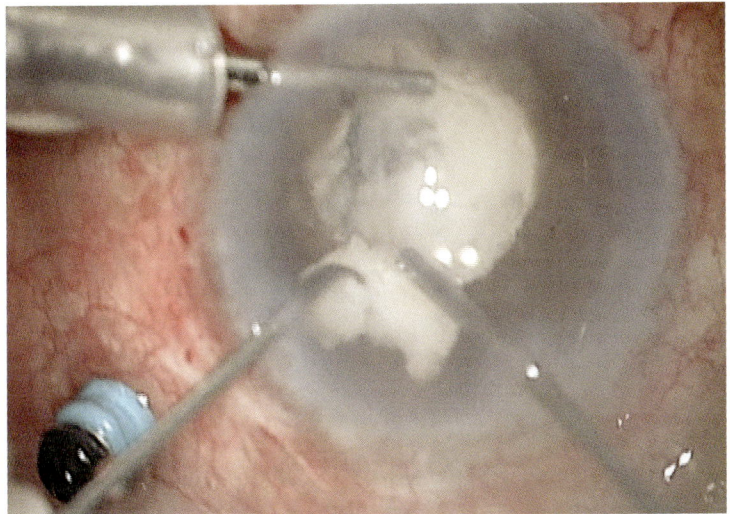

Fig. 11.5 Cutting freed thick exudates with the cutter bimanually.

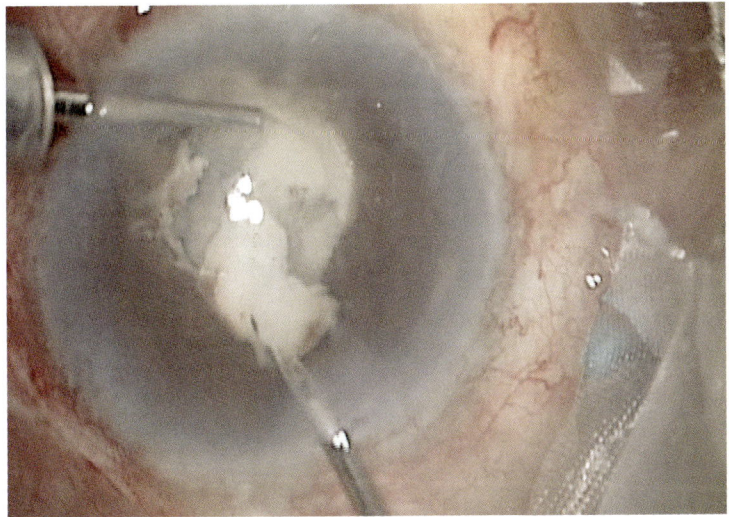

Fig. 11.6 Exudate being prolapsed out through the limbus-based incision with forceps.

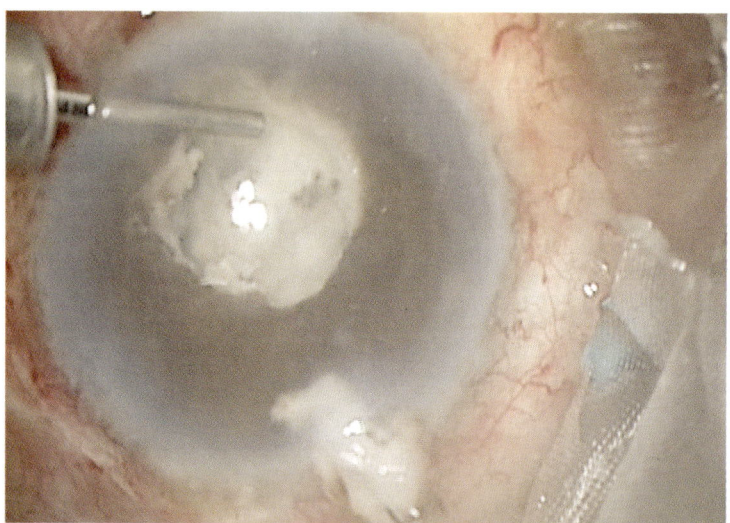

Fig. 11.7 Exudate externalized through limbus.

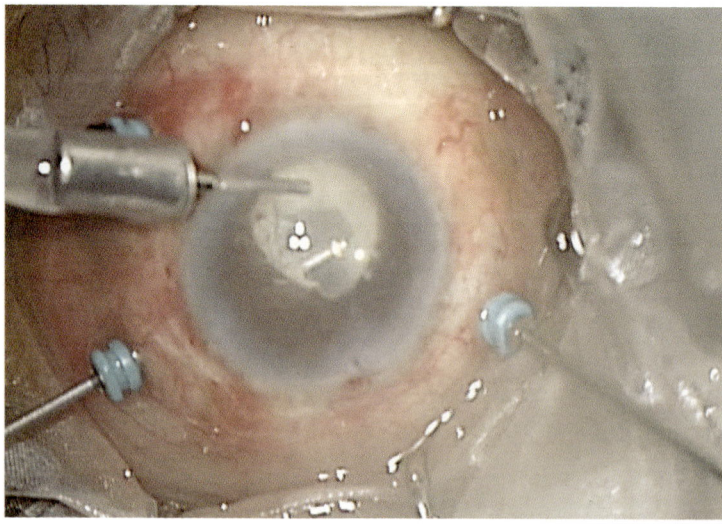

Fig. 11.8 Exudates being removed from the posterior surface of the intraocular lens with cutter.

- *Microbial sample*: After introducing the cutter, the first requirement is to collect an undiluted sample of the infected vitreous. This is achieved by connecting the aspirating end of the cutter to a syringe. A 0.2-mL sample is adequate and may be collected under manual suction with low-cut setting.

- *Vitrectomy*: Vitrectomy (**Figs. 11.9** and **11.10**) should be done at high cut rates and lowest possible suction to avoid traction on the cortical vitreous which is very sticky and adherent to the retina. Also, the retina may be necrotic and atrophic and hence prone to iatrogenic breaks, and the slightest of tractions may be disastrous. One should be absolutely sure of the tissue being dissected, as, in severe/chronic infections, the retinal vessels may be atrophic or absent altogether. Giant retinal tears have been known to be created for this reason. Complete vitrectomy is not

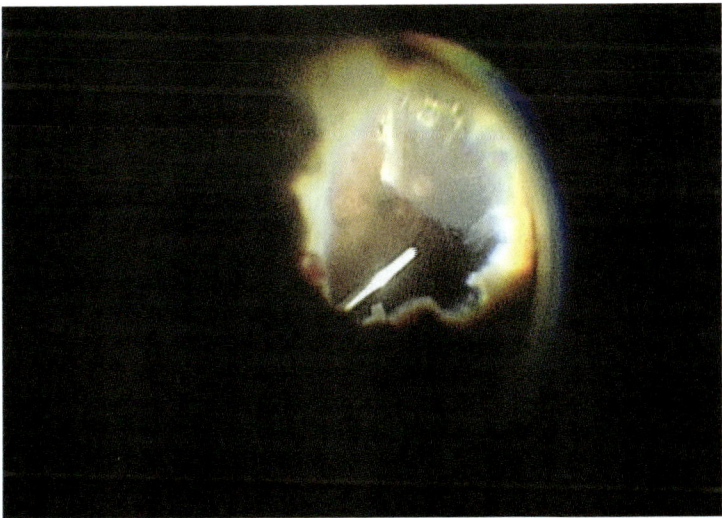

Fig. 11.9 Infusion cannula reinserted into the vitreous cavity. Slow core vitrectomy (note the yellow-colored exudates).

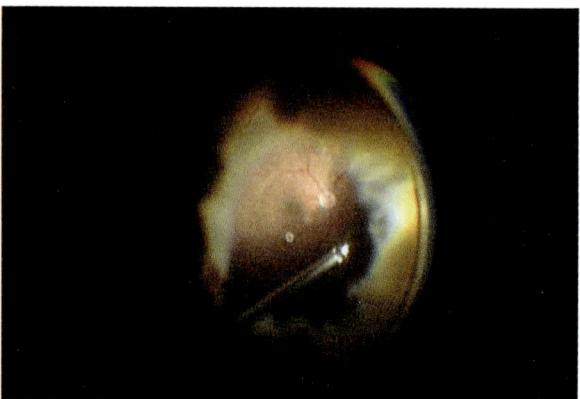

Fig. 11.10 Posterior pole is now visible with remaining peripheral exudates.

the aim in these cases. Even the EVS proposed only 50% of vitreous removal. Hence, visualization of the disc and the posterior pole up to the arcades is enough, and peripheral dissection is to be avoided because of the risk of breaks. Inducing a posterior vitreous detachment is not the aim, as this again may cause unmanageable iatrogenic breaks.

- *Macular exudates*: It is not uncommon to find premacular exudates. These should be minimally tampered with, and only blunt-tip cannulas should be used. These exudates usually dissolve later by themselves.

- *Iatrogenic breaks*: Despite all the precautions, retinal rhegmas are known to form in endophthalmitis. These necessitate tamponading agents. Only low-power laser should be used, as the friable retina is at a severe risk of tearing and the breaks enlarging postoperatively.

- *Exudative RD*: The presence of RD in these cases does not necessarily mean a retinal break because subretinal exudation, whether infectious or inflammatory, can occur in endophthalmitis.

- *Rhegmatogenous RD*: As much as possible, safe vitrectomy should be done around the breaks and the RD managed as in any other case.

- *Silicone oil*: Oil is known to have antimicrobial properties. In cases of breaks/RD, it is recommended as the tamponading agent of choice after fluid–air exchange (FAX) (**Fig. 11.11**). One may choose to inject it if retinal status is doubtful or in severe cases with risk of postvitrectomy phthisis. The surgeon is advised here to be in favor of using silicone oil in slightest of doubts as the postoperative period is very unpredictable and postoperative RD is extremely difficult to manage because of severe proliferative vitreoretinopathy (PVR). Oil here not only decreases the PVR but also slows down the process of RD, so that proper treatment may be offered when the eye is quiet in terms of inflammation and visual prognoses is not compromised.

- *Antibiotics*: It is recommended to inject intravitreal antibiotics at the end of the surgery in lower than their original dose to prevent retinal toxicity.

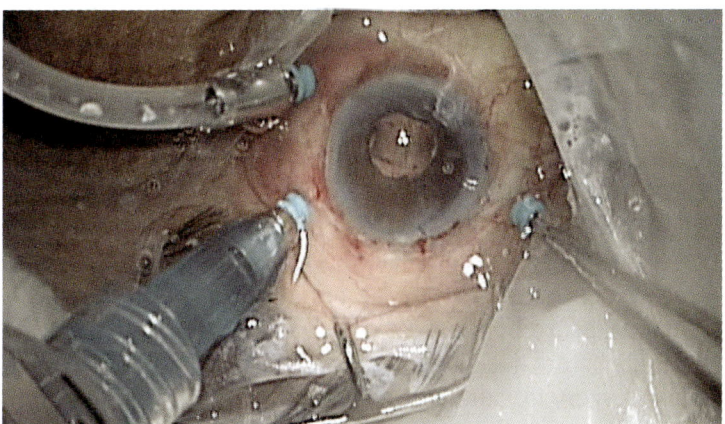

Fig. 11.11   Silicone oil being injected after fluid–air exchange.

In *P. acnes* endophthalmitis, it is advised to explant the IOL and the bag, which is believed to be the seat of infection. If the patient is unwilling for the same, risk of recurrence should be explained. In fungal cases, an abscess may be found. These should be debrided safely as much as possible, as these are the source for recurrent infections. In bleb-related endophthalmitis with severely compromised blebs, bleb excision may be necessary. Postoperative glaucoma is very common, and it should be specified to the patients. Vitrectomized eyes with endophthalmitis behave very badly despite vitreous lavage; silicone oil should be injected to avoid the risk of phthisis.

Complications and Prognoses

Topical and systemic antibiotics should be prescribed to the patient. Similarly, topical and systemic steroids should be used judiciously but very carefully in fungal cases or epithelial defects. Cycloplegics should be given, as the initial days usually show severe inflammations. Even AC fibrinous membranes may form. One should not be alarmed, as these dissolve over a period of time. Although anatomical results may be achieved, functional results depend on the viability of the neurosensory retina and the optic nerve.

Subretinal and suprachoroidal cannulas are common complications, and further complicate a very difficult case. RD and iatrogenic breaks occur as explained previously. Postoperative severe PVR and RD are again described. Both glaucoma and hypotony can occur. Persistent epithelial defects and cataract can occur. An inflammatory course in the initial postoperative period is common. Recurrent infections can occur and should be managed medically before deciding for resurgery. As per EVS, 35% of cases need resurgery for different indications.

Surgical Tips

- ✓ Good preoperative management and judicious use of intraocular antibiotics and steroids
- ✓ Patient management of AC
- ✓ Use long infusion cannula and do not start infusion till absolutely sure
- ✓ Only safe and adequate vitrectomy to be done
- ✓ Silicone oil tamponade

Retinopathy of Prematurity

Brijesh Takkar,
Rajvardhan Azad, and
Shorya Vardhan Azad

12

12 Retinopathy of Prematurity

Introduction

Retinopathy of prematurity (ROP) is a vasoproliferative disorder occurring in premature infants. Although spontaneous regression occurs in 80% of the infants, some of them require some form of treatment. A timely laser can prevent stage progression, but still some cases progress beyond stage 4 and require surgical management. Surgery is a challenge and rarely rewarding in advanced stages.

Preoperative Assessment

Work-up: Clinical examination is difficult and should only be done in the presence of a pediatrician when the child is systemically stable. Corneal haze, pupil dilatation, posterior synechia, and cataract require special emphasis. Indirect ophthalmoscopy with scleral depression is necessary for diagnoses and charting the extent of the disease. One should remember to use the correct concentration of mydriatic eye drops for neonatal examination (phenylephrine, 2.5%; tropicamide, 0.5%). RetCam-enabled wide-field fundus pictures may be taken. B-scan sonography is helpful in understanding the funnel configuration and therefore in determining the anatomical prognoses. A flash visual evoked potential/response is helpful in assessing the retinal viability and optic nerve function. It may also aid in choosing the eye with better prognoses in the setting of severe bilateral disease. Ultrasound biomicroscopy (UBM) is invaluable in assessing the surgical space available behind lens and deciding for cannula placement in lens-sparing vitrectomy (LSV).

Preanesthesia checkup: As the surgery is planned under general anesthesia for a child already under multiple systemic stresses of prematurity and vulnerable to complications, it is advisable to have a pediatric intensive care unit backup and a skilled anesthetist.

Examination under anesthesia (EUA): EUA is the final answer to the choice of eye and decision whether to embark on surgery or defer it in a setting of poor prognoses.

Indications: Stages 4b and 5 usually require surgery, while stage 4a may or may not.

Parent counseling: This is extremely important, as the expectations of the parents may be very high. Parents should be explained the risk of poor functional outcome and also the anesthesia-related complications in preterm children. Parents should be informed that navigable vision may be the best possible expected outcome. A sympathetic approach should, however, be maintained.

Aim of Surgery

The aim of surgery is to free the retina of all adhesion. After opening the funnel with viscoelastics/blunt dissection, attempt is made to relieve the retina of all visible traction without causing iatrogenic breaks. If successfully done, tamponading agents are not needed, fluid-air exchange (FAX) is done, and retina is expected to take its normal position with time.

Types of Surgery

Vitrectomy is the modality of choice in ROP surgery today. LSV is preferred for stage 4 and for cases where adequate retrolental space is available (can be confirmed with UBM) in stage 5. Microinvasive vitrectomy surgery (MIVS) (23/25 gauge) can be done in LSV, while suture-supported cannulas of 20 gauge are preferred in stage 5 ROP. Surgery is done with irrigating plano-concave lens and pediatric wide-angle lens system. Pediatric speculums should be used.

Stage 4 ROP

- MIVS ports are made 1.5 to 2.5 mm from limbus depending on age, and usually LSV is done (**Figs. 12.1** and **12.2**).

- Infusion cannula may be placed on the nasal side considering the usual temporal nature of the tractional fronds and should always be checked before switching on the irrigation.

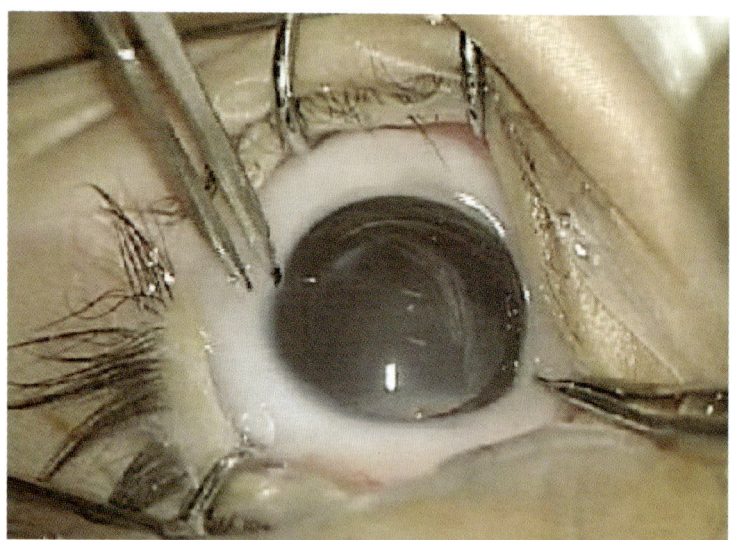

Fig. 12.1 Calipers for precise marking of port sites.

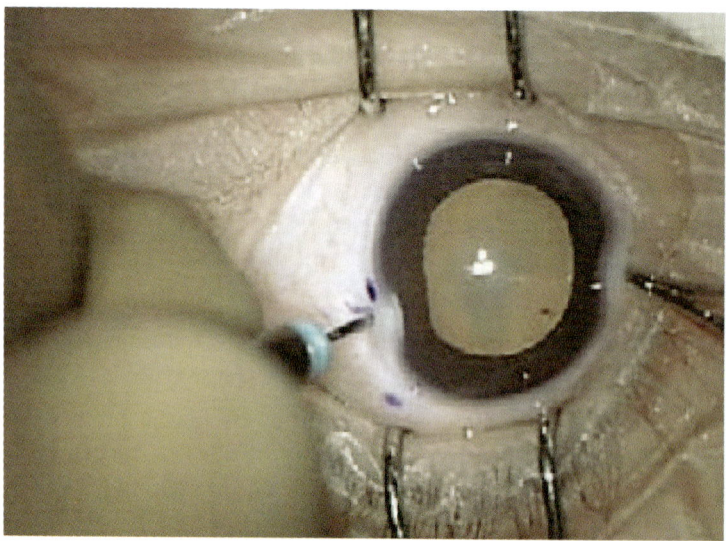

Fig. 12.2 Microinvasive vitrectomy surgery trocar being inserted.

- Vitrectomy is completed as in any other case, but posterior vitreous detachment is not induced.

- All traction is relieved with the cutter itself as anteriorly as possible (**Fig. 12.3**).

- Bleeders are cauterized.

- FAX is done (**Fig. 12.4**) and tamponading agents are usually not used especially in the absence of unsuitable configurations.

- Ports are closed.

Stage 5 ROP

- Lensectomy is most often required for stage 5 ROP, and surgery is very different from that of stage 4.

- Sclerotomy is made at 1 to 1.5 mm, and the aim is to place the infusion cannula inside the lens itself.

- Lensectomy is done and no capsular remnant is left to avoid recurrence of fibroplasia and posterior synechia.

- Differentiating retrolental fibroplasia from neurosensory retina is a challenge in itself, and dichotomously branching vessels are the best guide to decide dissection planes.

- Then the fibrous tissue is dissected with the help of bent 20-gauge needles/bent MVR knives (**Figs. 12.5** and **12.6**). Membranes are further separated from underlying retina with the help of scissors (**Fig. 12.7**) while avoiding undue traction on the underlying retina. Once a surgical plane is recognized between retina and fibroplasia, a 360-degree traction removal is performed with scissors/cutter (**Fig. 12.8**). Thus, blunt dissection is continued till posterior pole is visible (**Figs. 12.9** and **12.10**).

- At this time, viscodissection should be done while looking for unrelieved traction.

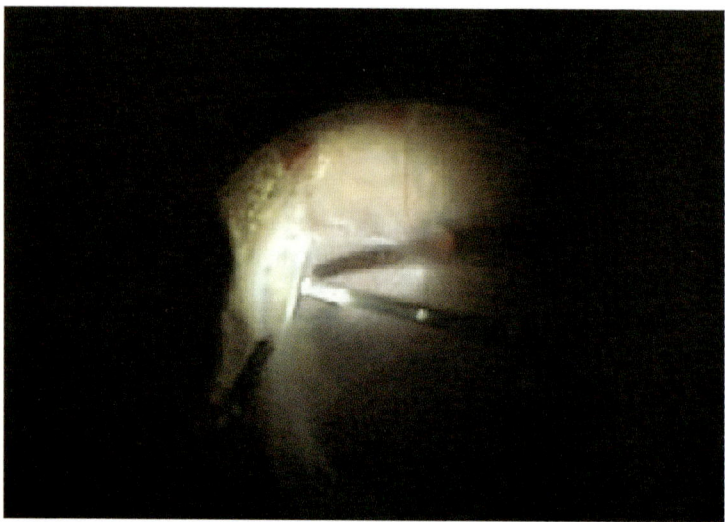

Fig. 12.3 Anterior traction being relieved with cutter.

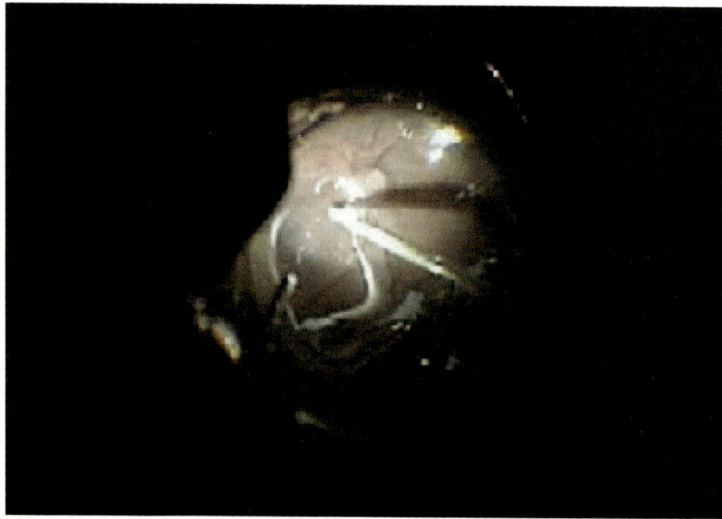

Fig. 12.4 Fluid–air exchange done.

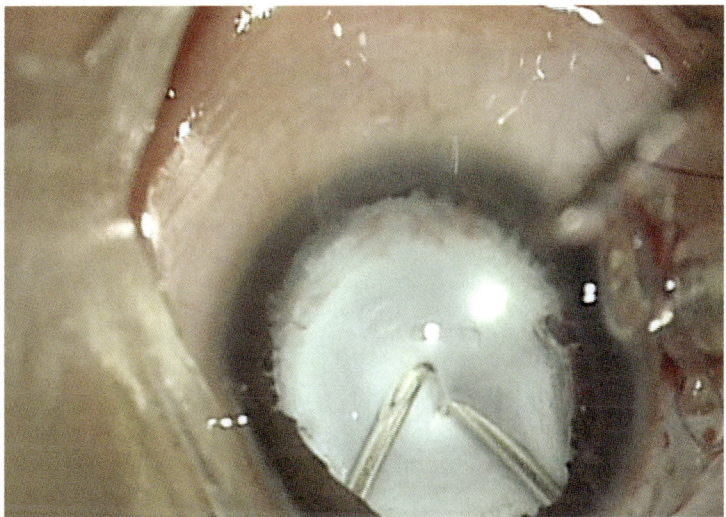

Fig. 12.5 Retrolental membrane being dissected with bent needles.

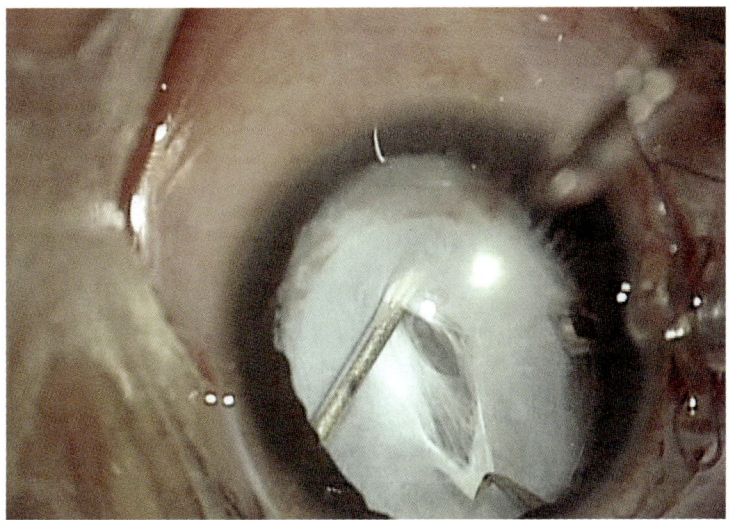

Fig. 12.6 Incision in the fibrous membrane enlarged.

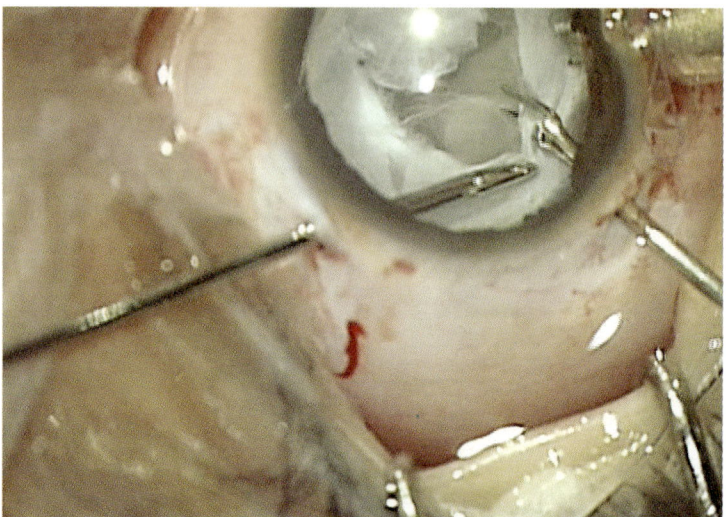

Fig. 12.7   Peripheral membrane being cut with intravitreal scissors.

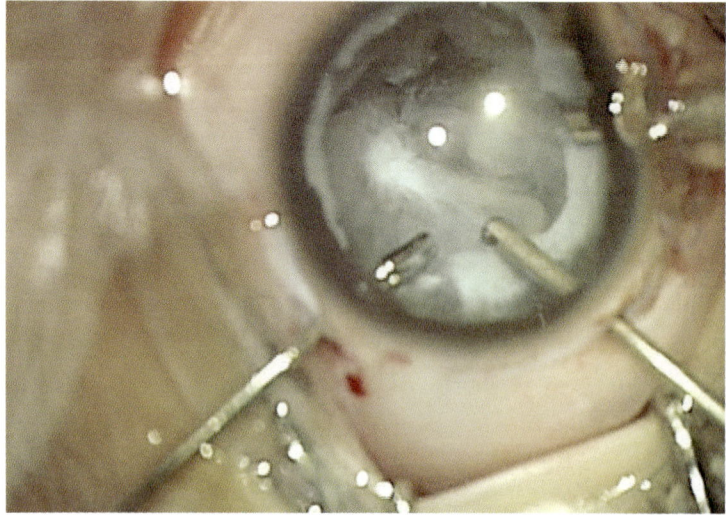

Fig. 12.8   Anterior traction relieved with cutter.

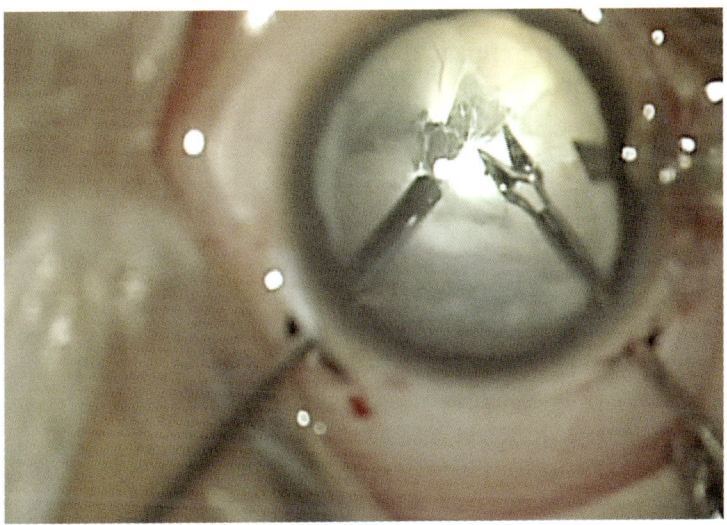

Fig. 12.9   Posterior traction being incised with scissors.

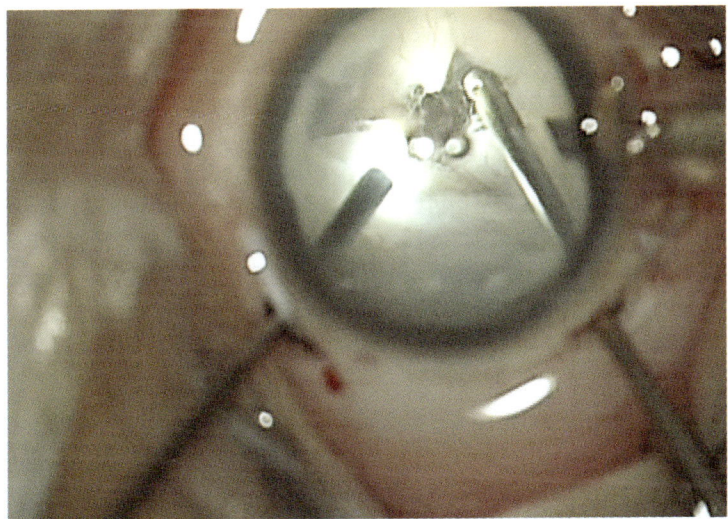

Fig. 12.10   Posterior traction being relieved with cutter till posterior
pole seen.

- Subsequently discovered membranes are then separated from retina to remove all traction, and scar tissue is dissected.
- Bleeders are diathermized and FAX done.
- Ports are closed.

Complications and Prognoses

Vascular fronds, if active, can lead to torrential uncontrolled bleeding during surgery, while regressed fronds are often unrelenting and very firmly adherent to the underlying neurosensory retina. Hence, iatrogenic breaks may form even during most meticulous and patient surgeries, which can enlarge as the infant retina is highly elastic. Subretinal bleeds may occur and oil tamponade may be needed. The retrolental fibroplasia may necessitate a lensectomy. Rarely, corneal haze and shallow anterior chamber can hinder the optical media required for vitrectomy.

After the surgery, it takes 6 weeks to 3 months before the retina falls back to take its position. Vision exercises are started only after the final settlement of retina. Monitoring has to be done for refractive error, glaucoma, and other complications of vitrectomy. Studies have shown close to 90% success rate in stage 4A ROP with LSV and nearly 75% for vitrectomy in stage 4B ROP. Stage 4B/5 cases requiring lensectomy do variably, with open funnel cases having reattachment in 50% of cases and closed funnel cases having reattachment in 25% of cases. Resurgeries are done for cases which have done well before but later developed complications.

Visually, results are very unpredictable; generally, LSV does better and even 20/20 results have been seen in stage 4A cases. It is better to do earliest possible intervention to avoid amblyopia than waiting for spontaneous vascular involution.

Surgical Tips

- ✓ Prudent case selection
- ✓ Entry point and direction of instrumentation are extremely important
- ✓ LSV for stage 4 and lensectomy for stage 5 usually
- ✓ Iatrogenic breaks have to be avoided
- ✓ Bleeding can occur from vascular tissue; residual blood should not be left
- ✓ Complete lensectomy is to be done to avoid recurrent proliferation, which is common in ROP

Complications of Pars Plana Vitrectomy

Brijesh Takkar and
Shorya Vardhan Azad

13

13 Complications of Pars Plana Vitrectomy

Introduction

With the evolution of newer and safer vitrectomy techniques, complication rates have decreased considerably. But still one may encounter these rarely, and managing such complications makes the surgeon wholesome and complete. However, before discussing the complications, we shall discuss the maintenance of clear media, which in turn checks the complication rate itself.

Maintaining the Media

Before beginning the procedure, the team should examine the microscope, wide-angle system, contact lens/Landers lens, or BIOME system for clarity. Optically clear cornea, lens, and a well-dilated pupil are essential for the best outcomes.

Cornea

Apart from inherent corneal opacification of the case, one should remember that intensive preoperative use of mydriatic drops itself can lead to transient corneal edema. Similarly, use of poor irrigating solutions can also cause corneal haze. Direct insult to the corneal epithelium by a sharp instrument can cause a small epithelium defect, which can again lead to epithelial edema due to hydration during the use of irrigating contact lens. Similarly, high intraocular pressure (IOP) can also lead to corneal edema. A previously predisposed cornea is more vulnerable to edema. Usually, intraoperative haze is epithelial and it is best to prevent them accordingly.

If edema is hampering, the surgeon should first try gentle stream rolling of the corneal surface, which often helps in decreasing epithelial edema. If this does not work, scraping of epithelium becomes essential. This can be performed with blunt instruments such as iris repositor while the assistant keeps the surface hydrated. One should only clear the central area and not scrape excessively. Also remember not to penetrate the basement membrane, as it can lead to irreversible opacities. One should avoid scraping epithelium in diabetics, as they have a compromised healing process.

Management of iatrogenic epithelial defects is essentially the same. One may encounter persistent epithelial defects which may require more careful follow-up with epithelial debridement, avoiding epithelial unfriendly medicine, using artificial tears and soft contact lenses. Prolonged pad-bandage may be needed.

Postoperative corneal decompensation can also occur, and it is managed as pseudophakic bullous keratopathy (PBK).

Lens

The most common lenticular problem is the development of lenticular opacity or cataract. It may be due to mechanical/instrument-related trauma or turbulence generated by the infusion cannula intraoperatively. One must be careful with regard to the position of sclerotomies and the direction of insertion of instruments in the globe in phakic patients. The surgeon must take optimum precautions; in case such a complication occurs during surgery, one must assess if the opacity is significant and located centrally enough to obstruct optical media. In that case, the surgeon may have to perform a lensectomy, phacoemulsification, or phacofragmentation depending on the age and sclerotic changes in the nucleus. Postoperatively, the tamponading agent, metabolic changes, and drugs may cause or hasten progression of previously noted cataract. Fluid-air exchange (FAX) and turbulent infusion are known to cause early postoperative fern-like or feathery cataract especially in diabetics, which is often transient but sometimes permanent. Rarely, lens subluxation may occur or may be enhanced due to poor instrumentation.

Miosis

This is a rather frustrating problem that may occur during the surgery. It may be caused by iris fatigue, mechanical irritation to the pupil, and pressure changes. This problem can be avoided to some extent by starting the patient on long-acting cycloplegics in the preoperative period (if not contraindicated) and using adrenaline in the infusion fluid. The surgeon can try using intracameral adrenaline, viscoelastics, proline sutures (Eckhardt's technique), and iris hooks.

Retinal Complications

Sclerotomy Related

Apart from mechanical damage to lens, zonules, and ciliary body, a wrongly placed sclerotomy can cause port-site retinal dialysis or vitreous base avulsion. Hypotonous eyes with or without clinically visible choroidal detachment are prone to suprachoroidal insertion of cannula. In such a case, the surgeon may opt to postpone surgery and give steroids. The cannula should be placed in an area where choroidal detachment is either minimal or absent. One may inject balanced salt solution/viscoelastics to increase the IOP before creating the sclerotomy. The best option, if possible, is a 6-mm 20-gauge cannula and should always be switched on under direct visualization.

Sometimes bleeding from sclerotomy sites may occur and may be very annoying. Usually, application of surface diathermy suffices. Uncontrolled intraocular bleeding may require a change of the sclerotomy site.

Port-Site Incarceration

Incarceration of vitreous or retina in the sclerotomy site is a disastrous complication if not recognized early. Early signs include tented-up vitreous toward the ports (both active and passive ports), and in some cases one may see the retina prolapsing out of the ports or the instruments may enter the subretinal space. The best way to prevent port-site incarceration is a meticulous port-site vitrectomy and avoiding insertion of heavy liquids in the eye before adequate vitrectomy. Recurrent movement of instruments across the ports should be avoided and anterior proliferative vitreoretinopathy (PVR) should be carefully dealt with. Still if such an event occurs, the surgeon should act swiftly by decreasing the IOP and guiding the retina inside with blunt instruments. The surgeon should cut the vitreous prolapsed at the port externally or enter through the opposite port and perform nontraumatic port-site vitrectomy from inside. Usually, this relieves the incarceration. Lastly, retinectomy may be required to solve the complication. With the advent of microinvasive vitrectomy surgery, such complications are rare, and even if they occur, they are less severe.

Retinal Tears

Iatrogenic tears are common bugbears and occur either due to direct retinal trauma or secondary to vitreous traction. These occur especially while peeling the epiretinal membrane, using high suction during peripheral vitrectomy, direct instrument touch, or large instruments such as foreign body forceps and fragmatomes, where even giant retinal tears (GRTs) can occur. Prevention by keeping low suction and high cut rates and directing the cutting edge away from retina is the best management option. Still if the retina gets stuck in the cutter, the surgeon should immediately stop the suction and keep the instrument absolutely stable. Reflux switch should be used or the assistant may be asked to pinch the tubing, which relieves the vacuum. One must indent the peripheral retina to look for such small breaks, which otherwise may go unnoticed. If they occur, the vitreous surrounding them should be shaved off and then retina adequately lasered. In the event of retinal detachment (RD) in previously attached retinas, the patient should be managed as for any case of RD.

Hemorrhage

Vitreous bleeds may occur from sclerotomy sites or due to dispersion of preexisting blood or instrumentation-related damage to vessels. These should be managed accordingly and are usually easy to manage. A bleeding retinal vessel should be cauterized or the IOP increased or direct pressure applied with blunt instruments. Diathermy at the proximal bleeder should be done in case the bleeding persists. A bigger problem is managing subretinal blood. Perfluorocarbon liquid (PFCL) can be used to prevent posterior migration of blood. If subretinal hemorrhage is fresh, passive aspiration should be performed immediately through an optimally placed retinotomy. However, if it is allowed to clot, the surgeon would need to perform active aspiration with soft-tipped cannulas or the cutter itself (**Figs. 13.1** and **13.2**). One may have to use forceps for old blood. Instrument-related trauma, sclerotomies, or sudden hypotony can also result in suprachoroidal hemorrhages. The IOP should be increased immediately. Although external drainage may be attempted, it is extremely dangerous and unpredictable. It is best to wait for the hemorrhage to resolve by itself in the postoperative period.

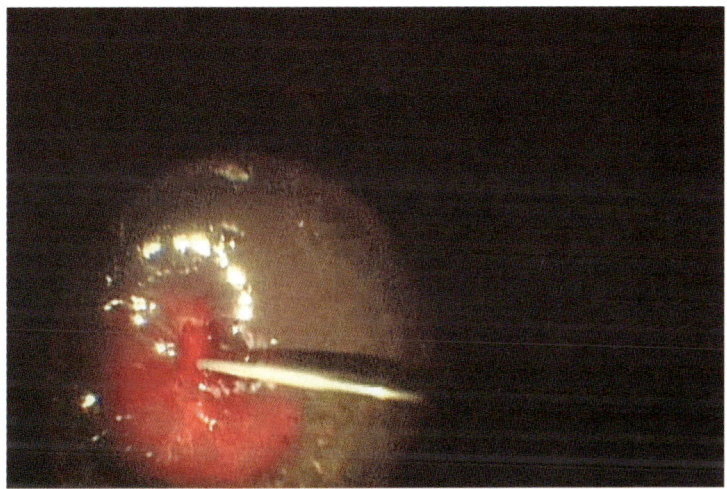

Fig. 13.1   Active aspiration of blood with soft-tipped cannula.

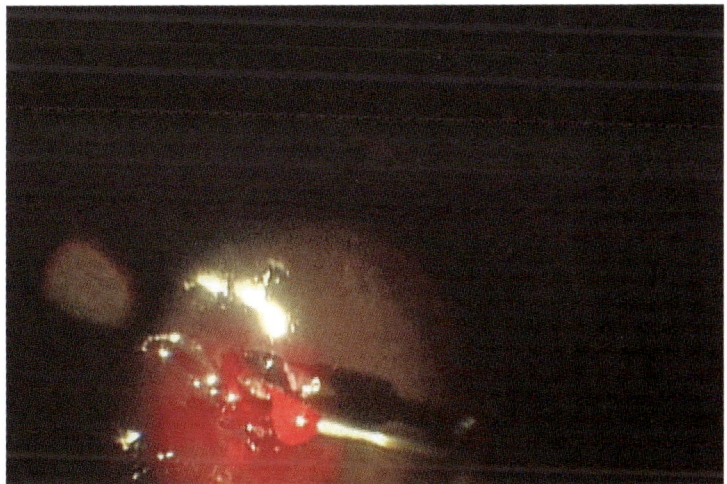

Fig. 13.2   Active aspiration of blood with vitrectomy cutter.

Rebleeds can occur immediately or late in the postoperative period, especially in diabetics or other vascular cases. Early on, they may be due to dispersed blood or port-site bleeds, while those occurring later are due to progression of neovascularization or residual vitreous contraction. Nonresolving cases may require vitreous lavage.

Subretinal Air

Air entering the subretinal space at the time of FAX is mostly due to residual unremoved traction at break sites. If such traction is adequately removed, air would usually come out of the subretinal site by itself and would allow the retina to settle. Another reason could be high indent at the break site caused by a scleral buckle which can be easily dealt with by loosening the final tie. If air persists to stay in the subretinal space, the surgeon can switch back the fluid to aspirate the air and may use PFCL for the same if necessary. Such situations warrant the surgeon to assess if the retina has become stiff due to PVR and hence may require retinectomy (**Figs. 13.3** and **13.4**). Small peripheral air bubbles, however, can be left alone as they get absorbed after a period of time.

One should remember that subretinal air is more likely if active fluid aspiration is done at high rate during FAX or if large breaks are present at the cannula site; hence, one should be prepared for this complication.

Endophthalmitis

It is very rare after vitrectomy as the seat of the infection has been removed. Intravitreal antibiotics and vitreous lavage may be done with endotamponade with silicone oil. The visual outcomes are usually bad.

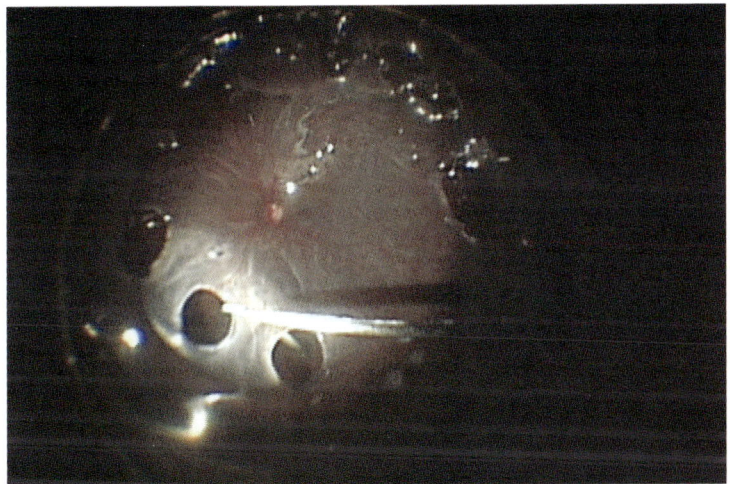

Fig. 13.3 Subretinal air despite relaxing retinotomies.

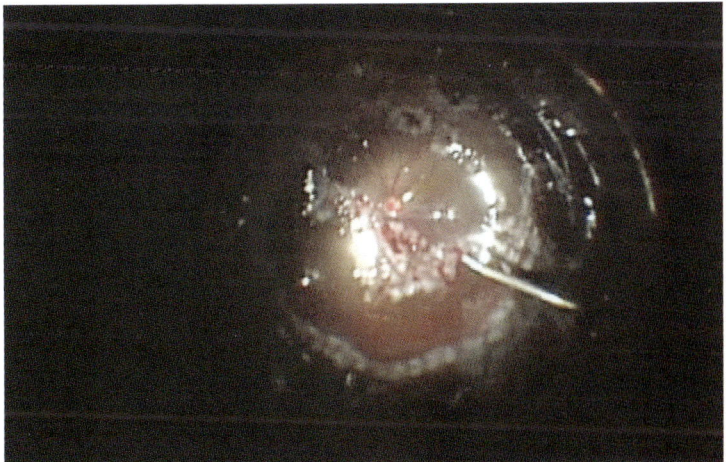

Fig. 13.4 Retina settled after retinectomy.

Sympathetic Ophthalmia

It is a rare complication after vitreous surgery. Few cases of sympathetic ophthalmia have been reported in the literature.

Recurrent Retinal Detachment

Proliferative retinopathy may complicate any case of RD and may lead to recurrent RD. Similarly, missed breaks, incomplete vitrectomy, residual hyaloids, improper positioning, and inadequate retinopexy may cause recurrent RDs. Preexisting PVR, high myopia, preexisting choroidal detachment, pediatric cases, severe vascular retinopathies, GRTs, colobomas, foreign bodies, and endophthalmitis are some of the cases predisposed to recurrent RDs.

Oil in the Wrong Place

Oil may enter the anterior chamber even in "adequate fill" cases in aphakic patients. In the absence of overfill, this oil usually reverts back to vitreous cavity with good positioning of the patient. In pseudophakic and phakic patients, the surgeon may opt for gentle aspiration in the absence of posterior capsule ruptures (PCRs) and zonular dialysis. If zonular dialysis or PCR is present, it is better to push this oil into position with viscoelastics rather than aspirating, as the surgeon may end up aspirating more and more oil. Small bubbles do not cause any problem in healthy corneas if oil removal is performed at the right time.

Subretinal oil may occur, which warrants removal with retinotomy and active aspiration. It is best to inject oil under direct visualization to avoid such complications. Subchoroidal oil may occur. In small quantities, it is usually harmless and can be milked out through an enlarged sclerotomy.

Choroidal Detachment

As discussed previously, it may be hemorrhagic or serous and is self-resolving usually. In the presence of CD, the fill of the tamponading agent should be titrated carefully.

Glaucoma after Vitreous Surgery

Glaucoma often complicates the postoperative period even after uneventful surgeries; hence, there is constant requirement of keeping the IOP under check. It is multifactorial, and management depends on the etiology:

- *Silicone oil glaucoma*: Pupillary block, overfill, emulsification-related, trabeculitis-related glaucoma may be caused by silicone oil.

- *Steroid-induced glaucoma.*

- *Pupillary block glaucoma*: It occurs in aphakic patients in which air, gas, or oil has been used. Peripheral iridotomy (PI) should be done inferiorly (Ando's PI).

- *Trabeculitis glaucoma*: Acute postoperative inflammation may result in glaucoma and lead to formation of peripheral anterior synechiae.

- *Encirclage related*: Compression of vortex veins caused by a posteriorly placed encirclage band can increase the episcleral pressure, resulting in glaucoma.

- *Neovascular glaucoma*: This can occur especially in vasculopathies when the lens barrier has been breached allowing the vascular endothelial growth factor (VEGF) to migrate anteriorly.

- *Angle-recession glaucoma*: This glaucoma may get unmasked after successful retinal reattachment.
- *Erythroclastic glaucoma*: It is a form of hemolytic glaucoma associated with leftover blood.
- *Malignant glaucoma*: It is very rare after vitreous surgery.
- *Open-angle glaucoma*: It may be precipitated or may progress after surgery.

Therefore, no surgical procedure should be taken for granted as complications may occur, and one should be aware enough to realize them at the earliest for optimum management. However, as "prevention is better than cure," the surgeon should realize which case is predisposed to which type of complication so that they can be prevented and patient counseling may be done accordingly.

Vitreous Substitutes

Shorya Vardhan Azad and Brijesh Takkar

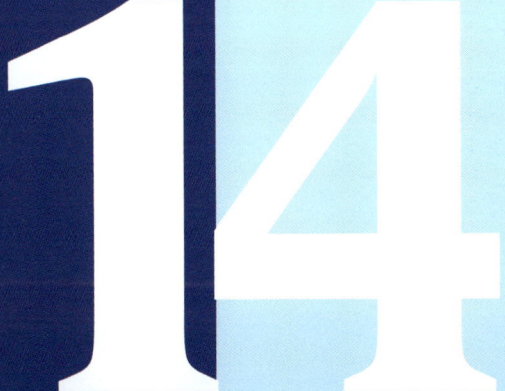

14

14 Vitreous Substitutes

Introduction

The use of intraocular vitreous substitute was first reported by Ohm in 1911, when he introduced air into the vitreous cavity to facilitate reattachment of the retina. Until recently, functions of the vitreous, apart from its mechanical and optical presence, are not well understood. Now we know that vitreous not only maintains the intraocular pressure (IOP) but also plays an important role in the nourishment of the eye. The ideal vitreous substitute should be transparent, elastic, and biocompatible as the vitreous itself. Vitreous substitutes can be divided into two groups:

- Conventional vitreous substitutes:
  - Gases: air, SF6, C3F8
  - Liquids: balanced salt solution (BSS), perfluorocarbon liquids (PFCL), and silicone oil (SO)
- Newer vitreous substitutes:
  - Semifluorinated alkanes (SFAs),
  - SO and SFA combinations

Conventional Vitreous Substitutes

Gases

Air

Air is mainly used intraoperatively during fluid–air exchange (FAX), facilitating retinal reattachment. It is easily available and inexpensive, but practical intraocular time is only 2 to 3 days, so it cannot be used for long-term tamponade.

Expansile Gases

Gases have highest surface tension (70 dyn/cm), which allows them to maintain good tamponading effect. Both SF6 and C3F8 have been used commonly in pneumatic retinopexy and in non-expansile concentrations for postoperative endotamponade. Depending on the percentage of gas injected, its intraocular stay can be varied. SF6 and C3F8 are commonly used in nonexpansile concentrations of 18 and 14%, respectively. It is eventually replaced by aqueous, avoiding the need for another surgery. Although gases provide excellent results, they can lead to cataract formation, corneal endothelial damage, raised IOP, and central retinal artery occlusion. Patients need to avoid change in altitude, as it can lead to sudden gas expansion. Gases cannot be used for long-term tamponade in complicated cases as well as in cases with extensive proliferative vitreoretinopathy (PVR).

Liquids

Balanced Salt Solution

Balanced salt solution (BSS) is the most commonly used intraoperative substitute as an irrigating solution to replace intraocular volume lost by vitreous removal. It has also been used as a vehicle to carry drugs for hemostasis, pupillary dilatation, and anti-inflammatory effects.

Perfluorocarbon Liquid

PFCLs are fluorinated, synthetic, carbon-containing compounds that are clear, colorless, and odorless. The most remarkable property of PFCL is the specific gravity, which is higher than that of water. Typically, the specific gravities range from 1.7 to 2.03. The intraoperative uses of PFCL depend on their higher specific gravity, because it enables the fluid to settle posteriorly, opening folds in the retina while expressing subretinal fluid anteriorly through preexisting retinal breaks. The direct toxicity of PFCLs and their tendency to induce inflammatory reactions limit PFCL use for a long-term tamponade. Commonly used PFCLs are perfluorodecalin, perfluorohexyloctane (F6H8), perfluoroperhydrophenanthrene, and octafluoropropane.

Silicone Oil

Silicone oil was proposed as a vitreous substitute in 1958 but was first used for ocular surgery by Cibis in 1962. SOs are polymers of polydimethylsiloxane. It is transparent, not miscible with water, and has a refractive index of 1.40. The viscosity of SO is designated in centistokes. Most clinical trials have used 1,000 and 5,000 centistokes SOs. Differences between the two are determined by the length of the polymer: greater the length, greater the viscosity. SO is the only substance currently accepted for long-term vitreous replacement. Recent studies suggest SO and C3F8 are preferable for long-term tamponade in complicated retinal detachments, and that SO may have advantages over C3F8 in certain clinical situations such as hypotony. It is preferable to use a SO tamponade if postoperative airplane or high elevation travel is planned, or with difficulties in postoperative positioning in children or adults with physical impairment. This makes it a more versatile replacement than air or gas. The time for the removal of SO is mostly around 3 to 6 months when the retina is attached and retinal traction is absent. Complications of SO are emulsification, corneal decompensation, band-shaped keratopathy, cataract, and glaucoma.

Newer Vitreous Substitutes

Semifluorinated Alkanes

Although PFCL has been used for endotamponade in cases such as giant retinal tear, long-term use of PFCL can set up significant high pressure on the choroid beneath the retina, so that the blood supply to the capillary system is impaired. The low specific gravity of SFAs (compared to PFCLs) is thought to produce less damage in this regard. SFAs are physically, chemically, and physiologically inert, colorless, and laser stable with densities reduced to between 1.1 and 1.7 g/cm^3. They have been seen to be well tolerated in the eye up to 3 months, but the main limitations are early emulsification and cataract formation.

Silicone Oil/SFA Combinations

Till now, no single agent has fulfilled the criterion for an ideal vitreous substitute. Also, none of the available agents provide adequate inferior tamponade; hence, by combining the SO and SFAs, it takes advantage of the high viscosity of SO and high specific gravity of the SFAs to produce a vitreous substitute with a good tamponade effect and lesser chance of emulsification. SFA is soluble in SO, but the solubility is dependent on the viscosity of SO and molecular weight of SFA. The higher viscosity of SO and the higher molecular weight of SFA make both less soluble in each other. The combination of both produces either a homogeneous clear solutions (heavy silicone oils [HSOs]) or separated solutions (double fills [DFs]), depending on the ratio of the two liquids.

Heavy silicone oil is heavier than water; it is a mixture of SO and an SFA producing a homogeneous solution. Newer HSOs are viscous, stable, and better tolerated, resulting in longer-time tamponade and lesser emulsification. Commonly used agents are Densiron 68, Oxane HD, and HWS 46-3000. Recent studies have shown good anatomical and visual outcomes with no emulsification up to 3 months with these agents. HSO works well as a long-term tamponade agent for complex retinal detachments involving inferior PVR.

DF was originally thought to bring about simultaneous superior and inferior tamponade. Since both SFA and SO are hydrophobic, it is possible to produce a single bubble with two layers, one layer providing upper support (SO) and the other providing inferior support (SFA). However, DF may not provide enough superior support, as it produces an "egg-shaped" bubble with pure F6H8 inferiorly and a lighter solution of F6H8 dissolved in SO superiorly; the bubble as a whole behaves as a tamponade that is heavier than water.

Choice of Agent

In most of our cases, we recommend doing FAX at the end of surgery to prevent port-site leaks and hypotony. Although the choice of agent in most cases is based on surgeon preference and experience, when in doubt, a longer-acting vitreous substitute is preferred.

In uncomplicated vitrectomies such as for vitreous hemorrhage, IOL drop, and nucleus drop, air is the preferred agent. Not only does it give the earlier-mentioned advantages, but it also keeps media clear and allows faster rehabilitation.

In cases like macular hole, epiretinal membrane (ERM), and small tractional retinal detachment (TRDs), gas like SF6 can be left at the end of surgery. Also in cases where iatrogenic breaks occur with no or localized RD with complete removal of traction, SF6 is preferred over C3F8.

In cases where long-term tamponading agent is required such as RD, RD with PVR, retained intraocular foreign body with PVR and vascular TRD, C3F8, and silicone oil are preferred. Current literature suggests that C3F8 should be the choice of tamponade in fresh RD with no PVR. We prefer long-term tamponade in advanced vascular cases to prevent rebleed and postoperative RD.

Postoperative Positioning

No positioning: In cases where air is the substitute, no positioning is required.

Propped-up: In patients with superior break with/without RD and residual vitreous debris/bleed, 45-degree propped-up positioning is advised.

Prone: In RD with multiple breaks, macular holes, ERM, and TRD, prone positioning is advised for at least 14 hour/day. Surgeon should explain that head should always be parallel to the ground while positioning.

Prone with foot end: In RD with breaks in inferior 4 clock hours and extensive inferior PVR, prone with foot end elevation around 30 degrees is advised.

Index